Global Dermatology and Telemedicine

Editors

VICTORIA L. WILLIAMS

CARRIE L. KOVARIK

DERMATOLOGIC CLINICS

www.derm.theclinics.com

Consulting Editor
BRUCE H. THIERS

January 2021 • Volume 39 • Number 1

ELSEVIER

1600 John F. Kennedy Boulevard • Suite 1800 • Philadelphia, Pennsylvania, 19103-2899

http://www.theclinics.com

DERMATOLOGIC CLINICS Volume 39, Number 1
January 2021 ISSN 0733-8635, ISBN-13: 978-0-323-83554-1

Editor: Lauren Boyle
Developmental Editor: Julia McKenzie

Dermatologic Clinics (ISSN 0733-8635) is published quarterly by Elsevier Inc., 360 Park Avenue South, New York, NY 10010-1710. Months of publication are January, April, July, and October. Business and editorial offices: 1600 John F. Kennedy Blvd., Suite 1800, Philadelphia, PA 19103-2899. Customer service office: 11830 Westline Drive, St. Louis, MO 63146. Periodicals postage paid at New York, NY, and additional mailing offices. Subscription prices are USD 416.00 per year for US individuals, USD 1,000.00 per year for US institutions, USD 456.00 per year for Canadian individuals, USD 1,055.00 per year for Canadian institutions, USD 510.00 per year for international individuals, USD 1,055.00 per year for international institutions, USD 100.00 per year for US students/residents, USD 100.00 per year for Canadian students/residents, and USD 240 per year for international students/residents. International air speed delivery is included in all *Clinics* subscription prices. All prices are subject to change without notice. **POSTMASTER:** Send address changes to *Dermatologic Clinics*, Elsevier Health Sciences Division, Subscription Customer Service, 3251 Riverport Lane, Maryland Heights, MO 63043. **Customer Service: 1-800-654-2452 (U.S. and Canada); 314-447-8871 (outside U.S. and Canada). Fax: 314-447-8029. E-mail: journalscustomerservice-usa@elsevier.com (for print support); journalsonlinesupport-usa@elsevier.com (for online support).**

Reprints. For copies of 100 or more, of articles in this publication, please contact the Commercial Reprints Department, Elsevier Inc., 360 Park Avenue South, New York, New York 10010-1710. Tel.: 212-633-3874; Fax: 212-633-3820; Email: reprints@elsevier.com.

The *Dermatologic Clinics* is covered in *MEDLINE/PubMed (Index Medicus), Current Contents/Clinical Medicine, Excerpta Medica, Chemical Abstracts,* and *ISI/BIOMED.*

Contributors

CONSULTING EDITOR

BRUCE H. THIERS, MD
Professor and Chairman Emeritus, Department
of Dermatology and Dermatologic Surgery,
Medical University of South Carolina,
Charleston, South Carolina, USA

EDITORS

VICTORIA L. WILLIAMS, MD
Assistant Professor, Department of
Dermatology, University of Pennsylvania,
Philadelphia, Pennsylvania, USA

CARRIE L. KOVARIK, MD
Professor, Department of Dermatology,
University of Pennsylvania, Philadelphia,
Pennsylvania, USA

AUTHORS

AMY K. FORRESTEL, MD
Department of Dermatology, University of
Pennsylvania, Philadelphia, Pennsylvania,
USA; Botswana UPenn Partnership,
Gaborone, Botswana

DEVON E. McMAHON, BA
Department of Dermatology, Massachusetts
General Hospital, Harvard Medical School,
Boston, Massachusetts, USA

RODERICK J. HAY, DM FRCP
The International Foundation for
Dermatology, The St John's Institute of
Dermatology, King's College London,
London, United Kingdom

ROSALYNN Z. CONIC, MD
Department of Dermatology, Case Western
Reserve University, Cleveland, Ohio, USA

ELLEN E. ANSHELEVICH, BA
Research Assistant, Department of
Dermatology, Perelman School of Medicine,
University of Pennsylvania, Philadelphia,
Pennsylvania, USA

KINGSLEY B. ASIEDU, MD, MPH
Department of Control of Neglected Tropical
Diseases, World Health Organization, Geneva,
Switzerland

AILEEN Y. CHANG, MD
Academic Model Providing Access to
Healthcare (AMPATH), Eldoret, Kenya;
Assistant Clinical Professor of Dermatology,
University of California, San Francisco School
of Medicine, San Francisco, California, USA

TIFFANY CHAO, BS
Medical Student, University of California, Irvine
School of Medicine, Irvine, California, USA

SARAH J. COATES, MD
Academic Model Providing Access to
Healthcare (AMPATH), Eldoret, Kenya;
Department of Dermatology, University of
California, San Francisco School of Medicine,
San Francisco, California, USA

MARC CORBACHO-MONNÉ, MD
Fight AIDS and Infectious Diseases
Foundation, Badalona, Spain

MEELOD DANESHVAR, MD
Resident Physician, Department of Surgery, UCSF Fresno Medical Center, Fresno, California, USA

ISABEL MARÍA DEL PILAR CASAS, MD
Professor of Dermatology, Comahue National University Faculty of Medicine, Director of Dermatologia, Comunitaria Argentina, Dermatologist at Hospital Provincial Dr. Ramón Carrillo, San Martin de los Andes Public Hospital, Neuquén, Patagonia, Argentina

HUITING DONG, MD, DMSc
Clinical Professor, Department of Dermatology, The First Affiliated Hospital, Zhengzhou University, Zhengzhou, China

SARA L. FLETCHER, PharmD, MPH
Pharmacy and Therapeutics Clinical Coordinator, Drug Use Research and Management, Oregon State University College of Pharmacy, Corvallis, Oregon, USA; Portland, Oregon, USA

ESTHER E. FREEMAN, MD, PhD
Department of Dermatology, Massachusetts General Hospital, Harvard Medical School, Boston, Massachusetts, USA; University of Miami Miller School of Medicine, Miami, Florida, USA

LUCINDA CLAIRE FULLER, MA, FRCP
Chelsea and Westminster NHS Foundation Trust, The International Foundation for Dermatology, London, United Kingdom

CAMILA G-BEIRAS, PhD
Fight AIDS and Infectious Diseases Foundation, Badalona, Spain

SEYEDALI GHAEMI, MD
Resident, Department of Dermatology, The First Affiliated Hospital, Zhengzhou University, Zhengzhou, China

DAMIANI GIOVANNI, MD
Clinical Dermatology, IRCCS Istituto Ortopedico Galeazzi, Department of Biomedical, Surgical and Dental Sciences, University of Milan, Milan, Italy

ADARSH KUMAR JHA, MBBS
Medical Officer, DI Skin Health and Referral Center P Ltd, Kathmandu, Nepal

ANIL KUMAR JHA, MD, FRCP
Founding Executive Chairman, DI Skin Health and Referral Center P Ltd, Kathmandu, Nepal

DONGKYUN KANG, PhD
University of Arizona, Tucson, Arizona, USA

RAKHI KARWA, PharmD
Academic Model Providing Access to Healthcare (AMPATH), Eldoret, Kenya; Associate Clinical Professor of Pharmacy Practice, Purdue University College of Pharmacy, West Lafayette, Indiana, USA; Indianapolis, Indiana, USA

LORATO KENOSI, MSocSci
Faculty of Social Sciences, Department of Psychology, University of Botswana, Gaborone, Botswana

ALEXIA KNAPP, MD
Department of Dermatology, HealthPartners Medical Group, International Foundation for Dermatology Migrant Health Dermatology Working Group, Saint Paul, Minnesota, USA

CARRIE L. KOVARIK, MD
Professor, Department of Dermatology, University of Pennsylvania, Philadelphia, Pennsylvania, USA

AJAY KUMAR, MBBS, MD
Head, Department of Dermatology, Manipal Teaching Hospital, Pokhara, Nepal

ALI LOTFIZADEH, MD, MPH
Director and Co-Founder, PASHA, Los Angeles, California, USA

TOBY MAURER, MD
Academic Model Providing Access to Healthcare (AMPATH), Eldoret, Kenya; Professor of Clinical Dermatology, Indiana University School of Medicine, Indianapolis, Indiana, USA

ORIOL MITJÀ, PhD
Fight AIDS and Infectious Diseases Foundation, Hospital Universitari Germans Trias I Pujol, Badalona, Spain

ASHKAN MORIM, MD, MPH
Director of Finance/Technology and Co-founder of PASHA, Los Angeles, California, USA; Resident Physician, Department of

Emergency Medicine, University of California Riverside, Riverside, California, USA

ANISA MOSAM, MB ChB, FC Derm (SA), MMed (Derm), PhD
Associate Professor, Department of Dermatology, Nelson R Mandela School of Medicine, University of KwaZulu-Natal, Durban, South Africa

KAREN ITUMELENG MOSOJANE, MBBS
Ministry of Health and Wellness, Gaborone, Botswana

MARGARET MUNGAI, BSN
Deputy Director Nursing, Clinical Services, Moi Teaching & Referral Hospital, Eldoret, Kenya

OATHOKWA NKOMAZANA, MB ChB, FCOpth (SA), MSc, PhD
Faculty of Medicine, University of Botswana, Gaborone, Botswana

HAJI PHILIP ODHIAMBO
Research Assistant, Academic Model Providing Access to Healthcare (AMPATH), Eldoret, Kenya

CHOON CHIAT OH, MD, MRCP, MSc
Consultant Dermatologist, Singapore General Hospital, Department of Dermatology, Singapore

LINDA OYESIKU, MPH
University of Miami Miller School of Medicine, Miami, Florida, USA; Department of Dermatology, Massachusetts General Hospital, Harvard Medical School, Boston, Massachusetts, USA

VALESKA PADOVESE, MD
Genitourinary Clinic, Department of Dermatology and Venereology, Mater Dei Hospital, International Foundation for Dermatology Migrant Health Dermatology Working Group, GU Clinic, Mater Dei Hospital, L-Imsida, Malta

SONAK D. PASTAKIA, PharmD, MPH, PhD
Academic Model Providing Access to Healthcare (AMPATH), Eldoret, Kenya; Professor of Pharmacy Practice, Purdue University College of Pharmacy, West Lafayette, Indiana, USA; Indianapolis, Indiana, USA

JENNY PUN, MBBS, MD
Lecturer, Department of Dermatology, Manipal Teaching Hospital, Pokhara, Nepal

AZIZULLO M. QOSIMOV, MD
Chief Specialist for Dermatovenereology, Ministry of Health and Social Protection of the Population, Dushanbe, Tajikistan

AASTHA RANDHAWA, MBBS
Medical Student, Manipal College of Medical Sciences, Pokhara, Nepal

ERIKA SAWKA, BS
Medical Student, Oregon Health & Science University, School of Medicine, Portland, Oregon, USA

AGGREY SEMEERE, MBChB, MMED, MAS
Infectious Diseases Institute, Kampala, Uganda

RUSTAM A. SULTONOV, MD
Resident Physician, Sughd Oblast Dermatology Hospital, Khujand, Tajikistan

SHERWIN TAVAKOL, MPH
Medical Student, Keck School of Medicine of USC, Los Angeles, California, USA

BHAGIRATH TIWARI, MScIT
ICT Consultant (Pro Bono), DI Skin Health and Referral Center P Ltd, Kathmandu, Nepal

GAIL TODD, BSc (Agric), MB ChB, FF Derm (SA), PhD
Emeritus Professor, Department of Medicine, Faculty of Health Sciences, University of Cape Town, Cape Town, South Africa

MARIA UBALS, MD
Fight AIDS and Infectious Diseases Foundation, Hospital Universitari Germans Trias I Pujol, Badalona, Spain

MARTÍ VALL-MAYANS, MD
Fight AIDS and Infectious Diseases Foundation, Hospital Universitari Germans Trias I Pujol, Badalona, Spain

PHELIX M. WERE, BS
Pharmaceutical Coordinator, Pharmacy Projects, Academic Model Providing Access to Healthcare (AMPATH), Eldoret, Kenya

VICTORIA L. WILLIAMS, MD
Assistant Professor, Department of
Dermatology, University of Pennsylvania,
Philadelphia, Pennsylvania, USA

XUEJIAO ZHANG, MD
Dermatology Resident, Eastern District
Branch, Beijing Emergency Medical Center,
Beijing, China

Contents

Regional Disease Patterns

The authors reviewed outpatients in a tertiary dermatology clinic in Botswana to expand knowledge on patterns of skin disease in this population with a high prevalence of human immunodeficiency virus (HIV). Approximately one-third of new and follow-up patients were HIV positive. Common dermatologic conditions included eczematous eruptions, viral and fungal infections, malignant neoplasms, vascular disorders, disorders of pigmentation, and mechanical/physical injury-related disorders. HIV has impacted patterns of dermatologic disease in Botswana, with Kaposi sarcoma being the most frequently biopsied condition. Given the shortage of dermatology specialists, resources should be allocated toward education and management of these most prevalent skin conditions.

Cutaneous ulcers in the tropics are a painful and debilitating condition that anchors people into poverty. In rural regions of the South Pacific, infectious cutaneous ulcers are caused mainly by bacteria, including Treponema pallidum pertenue (yaws), Haemophilus ducreyi, and polymicrobial ulcers. For this group of infections the term cutaneous ulcer disease (CUD) is proposed. Some infections can cause malformations on the bone that have a permanent impact on lives in endemic communities. Better characterization of CUD may help design diagnostic tools and more effective antimicrobial therapies. This review updates the knowledge of CUD and discusses optimized terminology and syndromic management.

Telemedicine/Technology

Telemedicine has the potential to deliver high-quality, affordable health care to underserved populations that otherwise would not have adequate access to care. The authors provide a snapshot of several telemedicine initiatives that have used information and communication technologies to connect patients with health care providers across various Asian countries with differing socioeconomic statuses. They highlight several factors thought to contribute to the success of telemedicine programs, such as financial sustainability, ease of use, and utilization of existing

Dermatology Education

health profession, any country, and at any stage of training. This article highlights the case for such an alliance; discusses existing opportunities and gaps in global health dermatology; describes the development of a new international alliance; proposes future directions; and reflects on lessons learned.

Tools for Dermatology Care in Resource Limited Settings

In resource-limited settings, point-of-care diagnostic devices have the potential to reduce diagnostic delays and improve epidemiologic surveillance of dermatologic conditions. We outline novel-point-of care diagnostics that have recently been developed for dermatologic conditions that primarily affect patients living in resource-limited settings, namely, Kaposi sarcoma, cutaneous leishmaniasis, leprosy, Buruli ulcer, yaws, onchocerciasis, and lymphatic filariasis. All of the technologies described in this article are prototypes, and some have undergone field testing. These devices still require validation in real-world settings and effective pricing to have a major impact on dermatologic care in resource-limited settings.

In Western Kenya, the burden of chronic wounds and lymphedema has a significant impact on functionality and quality of life. Major barriers to provision of care include availability, affordability, and accessibility of bandages. At the Academic Model Providing Access to Healthcare, dermatologists and pharmacists collaborated to develop a 2-component compression bandage modeled after the Unna boot, using locally available materials, that is distributed through a revolving fund pharmacy network. In partnership with nursing, use of these bandages at a national referral hospital and a few county facilities has increased, but increasing utilization to an expanded catchment area is needed.

Neglected Populations

"Currently, an estimated 70.8 million individuals worldwide are forcibly displaced due to war, violence, and persecution. Barriers to providing dermatologic care include the large number of affected people, their movement within and across international borders, security issues, and limited access to dermatology expertise and formularies. Screening protocols for skin diseases and sexually transmitted infections differ worldwide, raising the need for shared guidelines to assess migrants' health. This article reviews the literature of skin and sexually transmitted infections in migrants and displaced persons, highlighting the impact of social determinants on skin health and challenges faced in providing care."

The authors collected demographics and assessed the impact of vitiligo using Vitiligo Quality of Life (VitiQoL) and Vitiligo Impact Scale (VIS), followed by a focused survey and semistructured interviews with 22 participants in midwestern Nepal. VitiQoL and VIS scales did not indicate a large impact on quality of life; however, through interviews/focused surveys, participants expressed unhappiness/worry, problems in finding partners, securing employment, and social discrimination due to their skin lesions. These stressors are highlighted along with lack of proper physician counseling and vitiligo-related myths, which create psychosocial distress that may not be given priority in underdeveloped countries like Nepal.

People with albinism (PWA) in Africa suffer many challenges, including higher risk of skin cancers and deeply embedded stigma. We conducted interviews with PWA to determine factors influencing their quality of life (QOL) in Botswana. Physical concerns expressed included skin/eye health issues and limited access to health care. Psychosocial concerns included stigma/discrimination and myths/superstitions. Environmental concerns included barriers to personal development of education and employment, safety concerns, financial insecurity, and disability rights issues. Pervasive difficulty in obtaining equal rights to physical, psychosocial, and environmental health affected QOL. Education around albinism and disability rights are needed to improve QOL for PWA.

The concept of skin neglected tropical diseases has been widely adopted into the policy and strategy of various organizations, governments, nongovernmental organizations, and health agencies. By pooling information and resources across different diseases, whose primary manifestations affect the skin, it is possible to deliver integrated surveillance and control programs and promote advocacy and reduction of disability and stigma. A further key part of the skin neglected tropical diseases program is the development and validation of training methods for frontline health workers. Networks that allow those involved in this work to share and compare expertise are being developed through various organizations.

DERMATOLOGIC CLINICS

SERIES OF RELATED INTEREST

Immunology and Allergy Clinics of North America
Available at: http://www.immunology.theclinics.com/

THE CLINICS ARE AVAILABLE ONLINE!
Access your subscription at:
www.theclinics.com

Preface

The Growing Importance of Dermatology on the Global Stage

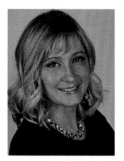
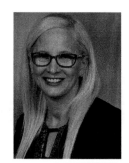

Victoria L. Williams, MD   Carrie Kovarik, MD

Editors

Historically, a significant focus of global health has been on life-threatening infectious diseases, such as HIV/AIDS, malaria, and tuberculosis. However, the Global Burden of Skin Disease project has provided eye-opening information to reinforce that skin conditions can contribute significantly to quality of life and disability. Skin conditions were the fourth leading cause of nonfatal disease burden worldwide, and the second to eleventh leading causes of years lived with disability globally in 2010.[1]

In addition to improving quality of life, the skills to diagnose and treat skin disease can also allow critical early recognition and treatment of life-threatening systemic diseases such as HIV. Because dermatology is less prioritized for allocation of resources, there is a smaller amount of funding available to support clinical care, education, research, and development of the field globally. Important questions in dermatology globally remain unanswered, and important work goes unrecognized because of barriers for publishing in major journals.

In this issue of *Dermatologic Clinics*, we have taken the opportunity to highlight a number of important issues in global health dermatology from a range of author groups representing diverse regions across the globe. We feature key topics in global dermatology that are lacking in the literature as well as notable examples of programs that will provide many key learning points. These topics include regional skin disease, telemedicine,

dermatology education, tools for dermatologic care, and neglected populations.

Skin diseases can have significant regional variation due to infectious diseases, genetics, culture, environmental considerations, and many other factors. We first look at regional disease patterns in Botswana, which have been heavily impacted by the HIV epidemic. Then, we review the current knowledge about cutaneous ulcers in the Pacific Islands.

A key tool for dermatology clinical practice in some resource-limited settings has been telemedicine, and we examine 2 local projects making an impact in this area in Tajikistan and Nepal.

The future of dermatology lies in the efforts we make today in educating the next generation of dermatologists globally. We highlight the International Alliance for Global Health Dermatology, a new organizational platform for global health collaboration that is making strides in connecting interested mentors and mentees and building international partnerships. We look in-depth into a successful community outreach project that has been increasing dermatology education for physicians and patients in Argentina. Then, we examine the current status of dermatology training programs in Africa, which suffers from a severe shortage of dermatologists for one of the densest populations worldwide.

We share progress that is being made in the development of innovative tools to improve dermatology care in resource-limited settings by

Dermatol Clin 39 (2021) xiii–xiv
https://doi.org/10.1016/j.det.2020.09.001
0733-8635/21/© 2020 Published by Elsevier Inc.

reviewing a low-cost local intervention for leg ulcers in Kenya and novel low-cost diagnostic tools for skin diseases.

Perhaps most important is that we highlight neglected topics in global health to which dermatologists in developed countries may not have been significantly exposed. We review the management of skin diseases in migrants and refugees, which is becoming more relevant in every part of the world in recent years. We examine how 2 visible skin diseases affect quality of life on 2 different continents. We first assess the impact of vitiligo on a Nepalese population and learn about the success of a local Vitiligo Awareness Campaign in decreasing stigma. Then, we take an in-depth look at the factors that affect the quality of life for people living with albinism in Botswana, which is of particular importance due to the unjust persecution and stigma facing this population across Africa.[2] Last, we review how integrated management strategies are improving the burden of neglected tropical diseases across developing countries worldwide.

We feel certain that with continued efforts dermatologists can make their voices heard to help others realize the important role we have in health care systems worldwide. This special issue is a small step toward disseminating the positive impact dermatologists are making globally. We are immensely grateful to all our contributors for making this special issue possible!

Victoria L. Williams, MD
3737 Market Street
11th Floor Dermatology
Philadelphia, PA 19104, USA

Carrie Kovarik, MD
3600 Spruce Street
2 Maloney Building
Philadelphia, PA 19104, USA

E-mail addresses:
tori22@gmail.com (V.L. Williams)
carrie.kovarik@pennmedicine.upenn.edu
(C. Kovarik)

REFERENCES

1. Hay RJ, Johns NE, Williams HC, et al. The global burden of skin disease in 2010: an analysis of the prevalence and impact of skin conditions. J Invest Dermatol 2014;134(6):1527–34.
2. Brilliant MH. Albinism in Africa: a medical and social emergency. Int Health 2015;7(4):223–5.

Regional Disease Patterns

Patterns of Skin Disease in the Context of a High Prevalence HIV Population in Botswana

Karen Itumeleng Mosojane, MBBS[a,1], Damiani Giovanni, MD[b,c,1],
Amy K. Forrestel, MD[d,e], Rosalynn Z. Conic, MD[c], Carrie Kovarik, MD[d],
Victoria L. Williams, MD[a,d,e,*,2]

KEYWORDS

- Epidemiology • Botswana • HIV-related skin disease • Dermatologic patterns • HIV-dermatology

KEY POINTS

- The high human immunodeficiency virus (HIV) prevalence in Botswana has had an impact on the overall patterns of dermatologic disease seen at a tertiary referral dermatology clinic.
- Approximately one-third of new and follow-up patients were HIV positive in the authors' cohort.
- Overall, eczematous eruptions; viral and fungal infections; skin neoplasms, including Kaposi sarcoma; vascular disorders; disorders of pigmentation; and disorders resulting from mechanical/physical injury were most common.
- Diagnoses that were more prevalent in the HIV population included Kaposi sarcoma, atopic dermatitis, flat warts, discoid lupus erythematosus, papular pruritic eruption of HIV, and lichen simplex chronicus.
- Kaposi sarcoma, squamous cell carcinoma, melanoma, lichen planus, and connective tissue diseases were the most common biopsy diagnosed conditions.

INTRODUCTION

Globally, the burden of disease for skin conditions is high. A systematic analysis for the Global Burden of Disease Study in 2017 showed that 3 of the top 12 most prevalent diseases worldwide were skin conditions and caused a higher burden of disability than priority health conditions like tuberculosis (TB)/human immunodeficiency virus (HIV) and cardiovascular disease.[1] Numerous studies have shown that the disability from skin diseases has far-reaching effects on the quality of life and performance of affected individuals.[2–7] Trained dermatologists are scarce worldwide, and resources allocated to manage dermatologic conditions often fall far short of what is needed, particularly in developing countries.[8–11]

In Botswana, access to dermatologic care is limited. The public sector has relied mainly on foreign dermatologists and trainees from North America and Cuba to staff dermatology clinics for periods ranging from 1 month to several years. To the authors' knowledge, there currently are 5 dermatologists working in the public sector and 4 in

[a] Ministry of Health and Wellness, Headquarters, Private Bag 0038, Gaborone, Botswana; [b] Clinical Dermatology, IRCCS Istituto Ortopedico Galeazzi, Department of Biomedical, Surgical and Dental Sciences, University of Milan, Via Riccardo Galeazzi, 4, 20161 Milan, Italy; [c] Department of Dermatology, Case Western Reserve University, Biomedical Research Building 5th Floor, 2109 Adelbert Road, Cleveland, OH, USA; [d] Department of Dermatology, University of Pennsylvania, 2 Maloney Building, 3600 Spruce St, Philadelphia, PA 19104, USA; [e] Botswana UPenn Partnership, P.O. Box AC 157 ACH, Gaborone, Botswana
[1] These authors contributed equally.
[2] This represents a previous affiliation when this research was conducted.
* Corresponding author. Department of Dermatology, University of Pennsylvania, Philadelphia, PA.
E-mail address: tori22@gmail.com

the private sector, all of whom are located in the 3 largest urban centers in the country. The wait time to see a dermatologist can be more than 6 months, and, for patients in rural areas, the time and cost of travel to a dermatology clinic can be insurmountable barriers. The main approach to compensate for the shortage of dermatologists has been to involve non-dermatologists in care and incorporate patients into the primary health care system.[8–12] In Botswana, a majority of patients with skin conditions are seen in local facilities by general practitioners with limited dermatology training or by traditional healers, which has been shown to cause poor outcomes.[9]

Information on the burden of skin disease is critically lacking in Botswana, which makes it difficult to appropriately allocate health care resources and train providers to care for dermatology patients. A governmental health sector report indicated that skin conditions were 1 of the top 4 causes of outpatient visits in the country from 2002 to 2006, but further studies on the epidemiology of skin diseases have not been conducted.[13] Dermatologic disease is particularly common and important in the setting of HIV, where systemic infections, malignancy, and severe inflammatory conditions frequently present on the skin. In Botswana, where the prevalence of HIV is the third highest in the world, access to timely and appropriate dermatologic care is of vital importance.[14] Understanding the epidemiology of skin disease in the general population and in HIV patients in Botswana is necessary to guide health care provision for this vulnerable population.

This study aims to describe the patterns of skin diseases in Botswana, with a particular focus on HIV-infected patients, in order to improve health care planning, guide resource allocation, and design educational programs to train providers to diagnose and treat skin diseases. This information also will serve as a baseline to understand epidemiologic changes in dermatologic disorders over time.

METHODS
Setting

The study was conducted in the dermatology clinic of the outpatient department at Princess Marina Hospital (PMH), the main government tertiary referral hospital located in the capital city, Gaborone.[15] Botswana is located in sub-Saharan Africa and has an estimated population of only 2.3 million.[16] It has recently been designated as an upper-middle-income country; however, significant problems with inequality of wealth, high unemployment rates, and a large rural population remain.[17] Access to basic health care in the government sector is free to citizens and consists of a tiered system of health posts, general clinics, primary hospitals, district hospitals, and 2 tertiary hospitals that provide escalating levels of specialty health care.[18,19] At the time of this study, the only specialized dermatology clinic available within the public health sector of Botswana was located at PMH.

Study Design

The authors conducted a retrospective review of new and follow-up patients seen in the outpatient dermatology clinic at PMH from January to December 2015. Data were extracted from excel files containing basic patient medical records, including age, gender, HIV status, diagnostic biopsy information, final diagnosis, visit type (new or follow-up), and treatment. Because individual patient information was not linked to visit data, it was not possible to distinguish which appointments were repeat visits by the same patient within the 1-year period. Visits that did not record these variables were excluded.

Visit diagnoses were first classified as single, multiple, or differential diagnoses based on the number/type of diagnoses given at each visit. Diagnoses that were listed only as part of a differential diagnosis were excluded from further subcategorization and analysis. The single and multiple diagnoses were divided into the major categories of inflammatory disorders, infections, neoplasms, diseases of vasculature, and other diagnoses (these included diagnoses that could not be classified under another major diagnostic category). These were further subdivided as follows:

- *Inflammatory disorders:* eczematous eruptions, neurocutaneous dermatoses (including pruritus and conditions related to chronic scratching, such as lichen simplex chronicus), vesiculobullous diseases, acneiform eruptions, follicular disorders, allergic/hypersensitivity reactions, lichenoid dermatoses, autoimmune connective tissue disorders, neutrophilic dermatoses, panniculitis, drug reactions, erythroderma, annular erythema, disorders of macrophages/monocytes, and other inflammatory disorders (including those that could not be more specifically subclassified)
- *Infections:* viral, fungal, bacterial, mycobacterial, and infestations
- *Neoplasms:* benign or malignant
- *Diseases of the vasculature:* vasculitis, vascular neoplasms (including benign vascular neoplasms, such as hemangioma and pyogenic granuloma), and other vascular disorders (including diagnoses, such as arterial ulcers, venous stasis ulcers, varicose

veins, Raynaud phenomenon, lymphedema, and elephantiasis nostra verrucosa)

- *Other disorders:* skin disorders that did not fit well into another category, including diseases of the mucous membranes, sweat glands, hair, nails, pigmentation and metabolism, genetic disorders, photodermatoses, dermatoses resulting from mechanical injuries/physical stimuli, transient noninfectious vesiculopustular dermatoses, and normal skin (indicating that the dermatologist could find no pathologic condition)

Treatments were divided into categories of topical, intralesional, systemic, surgical/destructive (including biopsy, excision, and destructive therapies of electrodessication, curettage, cryotherapy, podophyllin, or cantharidin), referral to another specialty, admission to the hospital, further work-up, and other.

Data were analyzed using Epi Info 3.5, version 3, and presented descriptively using means with SDs for continuous variables and percentage for counts. The institutional review boards of the University of Botswana, Ministry of Health Research Unit, and PMH Ethics Committee reviewed and authorized this study.

RESULTS

In this 1-year study, 3944 visits were reviewed and 2690 met the inclusion criteria. The patient population was 59.3% female, with a median age of 35 years (SD 19.26). Pediatric patients (<18 year old) were seen in 17.8% of visits and patients over age 70 in 1.7%. Regarding HIV status, 816 (30.3%) of the overall visits were with HIV-positive patients, and 169 (6.3%) had no reported results or had not tested in the prior year. Further sociodemographic characteristics of the patients are reported in **Table 1**.

Sixty-two percent of visits were follow-up visits (**Table 2**). Dermatologists diagnosed a single cutaneous condition in 2117 (78.7%) of visits, multiple conditions in 326 (12.1%) and provided a differential diagnosis in 247 (9.2%). HIV-positive patients did not have a higher frequency of multiple diagnoses or differential diagnoses but did have biopsies performed more frequently (51.2%) compared with HIV-negative (26%) or HIV-unknown patients (22.8%).

Table 3 displays a breakdown of the most common clinical diagnoses stratified by new versus follow-up visit, HIV status, and gender. The prevalence of disease categories was relatively stable between new and follow-up patient visits. Within the inflammatory category, eczematous eruptions were the most common specific diagnosis for new and follow-up patients. Under the neoplasm category, malignancies were the most common in new and follow-up visits. The infectious category revealed that viral and fungal infections were most common overall. Under the category of other disorders, disorders of pigmentation and mechanical/physical injury were most common.

In descending order of frequency, HIV-positive patients were diagnosed with neoplastic conditions most commonly (64.3%; 133/816) followed closely by diseases of the vasculature (53.2%; 25/816) and infectious conditions (47.3%; 112/816) (**Fig. 1**). Kaposi sarcoma (KS) was, by far, the most common diagnosis in HIV-positive patients in both new and follow-up visits (**Fig. 2**). Other common diagnoses for HIV-positive patients included atopic dermatitis, flat warts, oculocutaneous albinism, photodermatitis, lichen simplex chronicus, acne vulgaris, discoid lupus, herpes simplex, papular pruritic eruption of HIV, lichen planus, stasis dermatitis, genital warts, and psoriasis.

Table 1
Dermatology patient demographics

Patient Variables	Patient Characteristic	N (%)
Gender	Male	1094 (40.7)
	Female	1596 (59.3)
Age (y)	<1	75 (2.8)
	1–18	403 (15)
	19–40	1218 (45.3)
	41–60	819 (30.4)
	61–70	130 (4.8)
	>70	45 (1.7)
HIV status	Negative	1705 (63.4)
	Positive	816 (30.3)
	Unknown	169 (6.3)

Table 2
Dermatology clinic visit features stratified by human immunodeficiency diagnosis

Variable	Category	Total N (%)	Human Immunodeficiency Diagnosis, Positive, N (%)	Human Immunodeficiency Diagnosis, Negative, N (%)	Human Immunodeficiency Diagnosis, Unknown, N (%)
Visit type	New	1007 (37.4)	315 (31.3)	619 (61.5)	73 (7.2)
	Follow-up	1683 (62.6)	501 (29.8)	1086 (64.5)	96 (5.7)
Clinical diagnoses	Single	2117 (78.7)	624 (29.5)	1371 (64.8)	122 (5.7)
	Multiple	326 (12.1)	91 (27.9)	206 (63.2)	29 (8.9)
	Differential	247 (9.2)	101 (40.9)	128 (51.8)	18 (7.3)
Biopsy [a]	Not performed	2432 (90.4)	684 (28.1)	1638 (67.4)	110 (4.5)
	Performed	258 (9.6)	132 (51.2)	67 (26.0)	59 (22.8)

[a] Percentages calculated out of all new and follow-up patient visits.

Most patients received a single type of treatment or management recommendation (72.5%). Of 2985 treatments recorded, 64.3% were topical medications, 19.8% systemic medications, 5.2% referrals, 3.9% surgical or destructive therapy, and 0.4% hospital admissions (**Table 4**). A biopsy was performed in 9.6% of cases (258/2690). The most common histopathologic diagnoses were neoplasms, including KS (55.1%), squamous cell carcinoma (SCC) (15.2%), and melanoma (6.5%). Autoimmune and inflammatory disorders were also commonly biopsied (**Fig. 3**).

DISCUSSION

The current study presents, for the first time, the patterns of dermatologic conditions in a tertiary care hospital in Botswana. In line with previous similar studies performed in South Africa, Nigeria, and Ghana, patients were predominately female (59.3%; male-to-female ratio 1:1.5).[20–22] Reasons for female predominance likely are multifactorial; other investigators have proposed that women are more aware of health and cosmetic appearance and tend to seek early treatment of dermatologic conditions.[23] This slightly differs from a similar study in rural Cameroon, where the male-to-female ratio was 1:1.[24] In the authors' cohort, a majority of patients were young adults (median age 35 years; SD 19.3), as was the case in South Africa and Nigeria.[20,21,25] The relative scarcity of pediatric patients in the authors' study may be related to the tendency for most children to present first to their pediatricians who often can treat common skin conditions.[20,21,26]

Disease Categories

Overall, inflammatory diseases and, more specifically, eczematous eruptions, were the most common diagnoses in new and follow-up patients in the authors' cohort. This also is in line with studies from South Africa, Ethiopia, and Nigeria, which report eczema as the most frequently diagnosed skin condition.[20,25,27] In a dermatology clinic in Angola, eczema was the most common diagnosis in children under age 12 and acne in adults.[28]

Viral (40.7%) and fungal (46.9%) conditions were the most common types of infections, and there were very low rates of bacterial infections (4.9%) and infestations (4.9%) in the authors' dermatology clinic. These are similar to what has been reported in neighboring South Africa (dermatophytosis, 29.8%; , human papillomavirus [HPV], 9.1%; and bacterial and parasitic, 0.43%) and Angola (fungal, 19.6%; warts, 4.1%; bacterial, 1.9%; and parasitic, 1%).[21,28] Parasitic infections and scabies infestations are highly prevalent in many countries, particularly in climates that are more tropical than Botswana, such as Cameroon (onchocerciasis, 18.55%, and scabies, 2.82%), Ghana (scabies, 5.1%), Tanzania (scabies, 15.6%), and Ethiopia (scabies, 7.3%) as well as the desert climate of Saudi Arabia (cutaneous leishmaniasis, 4%).[22–24,27,29] Higher prevalence of bacterial infections have been reported in Central Africa, East Africa, and West Africa (Cameroon, 5.24%; Guinea-Bissau, 11.9%; Ghana, 17.6%; Gabon, 27.7%; and Rwanda, 22.7%).[24,30,31] One reason for lower numbers of bacterial infections in the authors' study may be that prior to evaluation in dermatology clinic, patients in Botswana typically see primary care providers who often trial oral antibiotics for anything that appears infected, as has been observed in Angola.[28] Other possible explanations for the differing patterns in Botswana include the more temperate climate, more sparsely distributed populations, and improved hygienic living conditions that may be due to the higher economic status of the country.[27,29,31,32] A study in Nigeria that

Table 3

Patterns of clinical diagnoses in patients presenting to dermatology clinic at Princess Marina Hospital

Diagnosis	New Visits, N disorders (%)			Follow-up Visits, N disorders (%)		
	Total	Human Immunodeficiency Diagnosis positive	Female patients	Total	Human Immunodeficiency Diagnosis positive	Female patients
All diagnoses	956	290 (30.3)	609(63.7)	1734	555 (32)	1203 (69.4)
Inflammatory	412 (43[a])	126 (43.4[a])	338 (55.5[a])	914 (52.7[a])	232 (41.8[a])	761 (63.3[a])
Eczematous eruptions	149 (36.2)	40 (31.7)	119 (35.2)	278 (30.4)	55 (23.7)	223 (29.3)
Acneiform eruptions	62 (15.0)	10 (7.9)	47 (13.9)	167 (18.3)	19 (8.2)	98 (12.9)
Follicular disorders	37 (9.0)	10 (7.9)	20 (5.9)	72 (7.9)	27 (11.6)	33 (4.3)
Neurocutaneous disorders	36 (8.7)	10 (7.9)	26 (7.7)	73 (8.0)	32 (13.8)	72 (9.5)
Allergic/hypersensitivity reactions	26 (6.3)	16 (12.7)	23 (6.8)	25 (2.7)	16 (6.9)	21 (2.8)
Autoimmune disorders	26 (6.3)	10 (7.9)	30 (8.9)	97 (10.6)	27 (11.6)	105 (13.8)
Drug reactions	23 (5.6)	11 (8.7)	17 (5.0)	14 (1.5)	6 (2.6)	14 (1.8)
Other inflammatory disorders	19 (4.6)	6 (4.8)	18 (5.3)	72 (7.9)	20 (8.6)	63 (8.3)
Lichenoid dermatoses	16 (3.9)	7 (5.6)	18 (5.3)	44 (4.8)	16 (6.9)	48 (6.3)
Vesiculobullous disease	7 (1.7)	0 (0)	8 (2.4)	33 (3.6)	0 (0)	33 (4.3)
Erythroderma	3 (0.7)	2 (1.6)	3 (0.9)	3 (0.3)	1 (0.4)	2 (0.3)
Macrophage-related disorders	3 (0.7)	0 (0)	5 (1.5)	19 (2.1)	5 (2.2)	24 (3.2)
Neutrophilic dermatoses	2 (0.5)	2 (1.6)	3 (0.9)	4 (0.4)	0 (0)	3 (0.4)
Panniculitis	1 (0.2)	0 (0)	2 (0.6)	11 (1.2)	6 (2.6)	17 (2.2)
Annular erythema	1 (0.2)	0 (0)	2 (0.6)	3 (0.3)	0 (0)	5 (0.7)
Neoplastic	88 (9.2[a])	53 (18.3[a])	68 (11.2[a])	119 (6.9[a])	80 (14.4[a])	108 (9[a])
Malignant neoplasms	59 (67.0)	53 (100)	41 (60.3)	94 (79.0)	71 (88.8)	77 (71.3)
Benign neoplasms	29 (33.0)	0 (0)	27 (39.7)	25 (21.0)	9 (11.3)	32 (29.7)
Infections	80 (8.4[a])	14 (4.8[a])	56 (9.2[a])	157 (9.1[a])	98 (17.7[a])	122 (10.1[a])
Fungal	38 (47.5)	13 (92.9)	23 (41.2)	40 (25.5)	17 (17.3)	23 (18.9)
Viral	33 (41.3)	0 (0)	29 (51.8)	105 (66.9)	78 (79.6)	92 (75.4)
Bacterial	4 (5.0)	0 (0)	3 (5.4)	7 (4.5)	0 (0)	3 (2.5)
Infestations	3(3.8)	1 (7.1)	0 (0)	4 (2.5)	3 (3.1)	3 (2.5)

(continued on next page)

Table 3
(continued)

Diagnosis	New Visits, N disorders (%)			Follow-up Visits, N disorders (%)		
	Total	Human Immunodeficiency Diagnosis positive	Female patients	Total	Human Immunodeficiency Diagnosis positive	Female patients
Mycobacterial	2 (2.5)	0 (0)	2 (3.6)	1 (0.6)	0 (0)	2 (1.6)
Diseases of vasculature	28 (2.9[a])	12 (4.1[a])	25 (4.1[a])	19 (1.1[a])	13 (2.3[a])	13 (1.1[a])
Vascular disorders	20 (71.4)	9 (75.0)	15 (60.0)	13 (68.4)	11 (84.6)	8 (61.5)
Vascular neoplasms	5 (17.9)	1 (8.3)	6 (24.0)	4 (21.1)	1 (7.7)	4 (30.8)
Vasculitis	3 (10.7)	2 (16.7)	4 (16.0)	2 (10.5)	1 (7.7)	1 (7.7)
Other disorders	348 (36.4[a])	85 (29.3[a])	122 (20[a])	525 (30.3[a])	132 (23.8[a])	199 (16.5[a])
Disorders of pigmentation	124 (35.6)	32 (37.6)	48 (39.3)	155 (29.5)	34 (25.8)	65 (32.7)
Mechanical/physical injury dermatoses	94 (27.0)	18 (21.2)	30 (24.6)	117 (22.3)	0 (0)	35 (17.6)
Genetic disorders	38 (10.9)	12 (14.1)	17 (13.9)	82 (15.6)	4 (3.0)	35 (17.6)
Photodermatoses	23 (6.6)	15 (17.6)	2 (1.6)	64 (12.2)	53 (40.2)	15 (7.5)
Disorders of the mucous membranes	15 (4.3)	0 (0)	9 (7.4)	15 (2.9)	15 (11.4)	9 (4.5)
Normal skin	13 (3.7)	3 (3.5)	2 (1.6)	10 (1.9)	0 (0)	3 (1.5)
Disorders of the sweat glands	13 (3.7)	0 (0)	5 (4.1)	10 (1.9)	0 (0)	2 (1.0)
Metabolic disorders	10 (2.9)	3 (3.5)	5 (4.1)	23 (4.4)	23 (17.4)	11 (5.5)
Nail disorders	10 (2.9)	3 (3.5)	3 (2.5)	8 (1.5)	4 (3.0)	5 (2.5)
Disorders of the hair	8 (2.3)	0 (0)	3 (2.5)	41 (7.8)	0 (0)	21 (10.6)

[a] These percentages are out of total column N; otherwise, all percentages are out of each individual category N total.

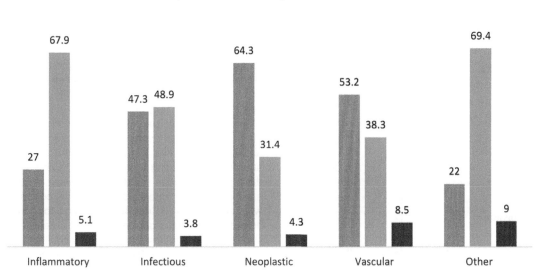

Fig. 1. Major disease categories for dermatology diagnoses stratified by HIV status.

investigated changes in the epidemiology of skin disease over a 30-year period showed that recent disease patterns more closely mirrored the authors' data: an increase in eczema, acne, pigmentary disorders, and warts and a decrease in bacterial infections and scabies.[25] The Nigerian investigators attributed this epidemiologic shift to urbanization and improved socioeconomic conditions.[25]

Within the neoplasm category, malignant neoplasms were more frequent, and KS was the overall most common malignancy. The top 3

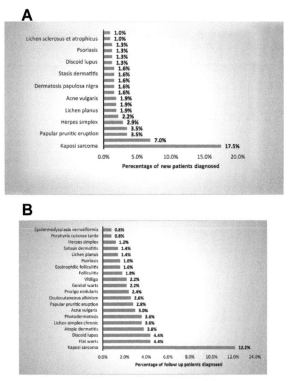

Fig. 2. Most frequent dermatology clinical diagnoses in new (*A*) and follow-up (*B*) HIV-positive patients.

Table 4 Summary of treatments for skin diseases over all dermatology patient visits		
Overall Treatments Total N = 2985	**N**	**Percentage**
Single treatment	2164	72.5
Multiple treatments	821	27.5
Treatment types		
Topical	1919	64.3
Intralesional	63	2.1
Systemic	591	19.8
Surgical/destructive	116	3.9
Referral	155	5.2
Admission	12	0.4
Further work-up	7	0.2
Other	122	4.1

diagnoses made by histopathology were KS (55.1%) (**Fig. 4**A), SCC (15.2%), and melanoma (6.5%). In the Northern Cape of South Africa, York and colleagues[33] reported the top 3 malignant neoplasms as SCC (45.4%), basal cell carcinoma (27.8%), and KS (6.5%). Similarly, KS and SCC were the most prevalent malignancies in a study from Tanzania.[34] In African populations, SCC has been reported as the overall most common malignancy and is associated more often with chronic wounds in these populations.[35] In

the authors' dermatology population, they have observed HIV-associated immunosuppression, HPV, and oculocutaneous albinism to be the major risk factors for SCC (**Fig. 4**B). The authors' histopathologic diagnostic patterns reflect both the impact of HIV on dermatologic conditions in Botswana and the intentional preferential selection of malignant or life-threatening conditions to biopsy. This histologic picture differs greatly with other countries in the world, where conditions, such as eczema, psoriasis, and lichen planus, are among common histologic diagnoses.[36] The time from performing a biopsy to receiving a pathology result varies widely in Botswana. A turnaround time of 4 weeks to 10 weeks is common, which drastically reduces its usefulness for conditions that require urgent management decisions, such as malignancies and others (vasculitis, vasculopathy, systemic infections, severe drug reactions, or blistering eruptions). Because punch and shave biopsy tools have not been obtainable locally, the dermatology clinic at PMH has relied on donations by visiting North American trainees over the past 10 years. If the histopathologic turnaround time were shorter, more pathologists with dermatopathology expertise were available, and supplies were continuously available locally, biopsies could be performed for a wider range of conditions, which could improve outcomes and increase our understanding of dermatologic conditions in Botswana.[22]

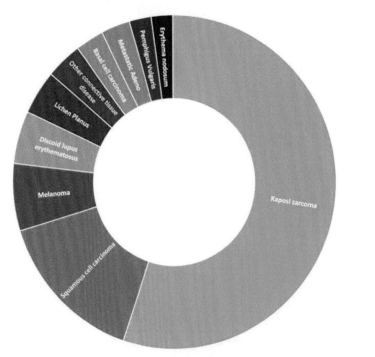

Fig. 3. The top 10 diagnoses out of all patients undergoing biopsy at PMC dermatology clinic.

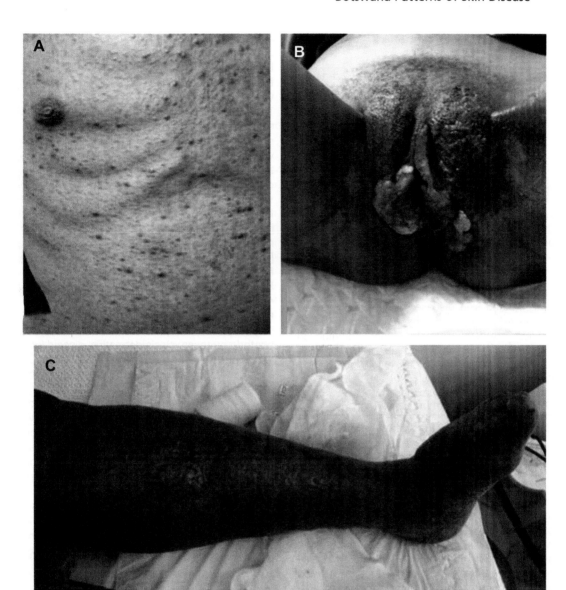

Fig. 4. (*A*) Disseminated violaceous papules of KS in an HIV-positive patient. (*B*) Multifocal exophytic labial masses in an HIV-positive patient with genital warts that have progressed to an invasive SCC. (*C*) An HIV-positive patient with chronic lymphedema of the left leg associated with KS that was treated with ARVs, chemotherapy, and radiation.

Within the diseases of vasculature category, general vascular disorders were most common, which includes peripheral vascular disease and stasis associated disorders like lymphedema. HIV is a known risk factor for peripheral vascular disease and the authors correspondingly noted a higher rate of the diseases of vasculature for HIV-positive patients (**Fig. 4**C). It is the authors' experience that a significant portion of patients in Botswana present with lymphedema secondary to HIV and/or associated with KS, which also has been reported by Santos and colleagues.[37] Worldwide, vascular disorders can cause an immense burden to health care systems due to chronic leg ulcers and lymphedema that cause recurrent infections, pain, and impair mobility.[38–41] Early recognition is key, because early intervention reduces the risk of long-term morbidity.

Disorders of pigmentation and mechanical/physical injury were the most commonly diagnosed within the category of "other disorders." Dyschromias were also commonly reported in South Africa and Ethiopia.[20,21,27] The authors'

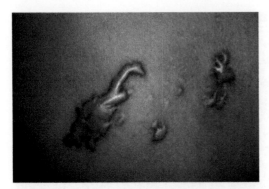

Fig. 5. Skin-colored polymorphous keloidal plaques that developed post-zoster infection in an HIV-positive patient.

study highlights a high frequency of physical injury–related skin disease, which encompasses diagnoses, such as keloids (**Fig. 5**) and scars. Keloids are known to be more common in darker skin types and were also reported at a high frequency in an epidemiologic study from Cameroon.[24,42]

Diagnosis and Treatment Patterns

Overall, in a majority of the authors' visits (78.7%), a single diagnosis was made through clinical examination or bedside diagnostic testing.[22,24,43,44] Topical medications were the most common type of treatment prescribed (64.3%), followed by systemic medications (19.8%), which is similar to dermatology treatment patterns reported in other developing countries.[22,24,43,44] Skin biopsy was performed in only 9.6% of visits, but it is the authors' experience that more patients could benefit from biopsy to confirm diagnoses. Due to the previously discussed resource limitations, however, the authors' clinic must triage biopsies for cases in which histology may significantly change management, when there is no response to treatment, or when there is concern for a malignant condition, as is the case in many other countries in Africa.[22]

Human Immunodeficiency Virus and Skin Disease

The authors' data confirm that HIV patients experience a significant burden of skin disease requiring specialized dermatologic evaluation. More than 30% of the dermatology cohort was HIV positive, which is slightly higher than the most recently reported HIV prevalence of 20.3% in the adult population of Botswana in 2019.[45] Botswana is striving toward the UNAIDS target of 90-90-90, in which 90% of patients should be

aware of their HIV status, started on treatment, and virally suppressed by the year 2020.[46] Encouragingly, 93.7% of the authors' dermatology patients in 2015 knew their HIV status, which is slightly higher than the national target. The top diagnoses in HIV-positive patients were similar for new and follow-up visits. KS was the most frequent overall diagnosis in 17.5% of new visits for HIV patients. As expected, within the top 20 conditions for HIV-positive patients were diseases that are known to be more frequent, severe, and atypical in this population, including infections (flat warts [**Fig. 6**A], herpes simplex virus [**Fig. 6**B], genital warts, tinea, folliculitis, epidermodysplasia verruciformis, drug reactions [Stevens-Johnson syndrome], HIV-associated inflammatory diseases [papular pruritic eruption of HIV (**Fig. 6**D)], and eosinophilic folliculitis) and a range of inflammatory or autoimmune conditions that can worsen with HIV (atopic dermatitis [**Fig. 6**C], lichen simplex chronicus, lichen planus, photodermatoses, stasis dermatitis, discoid lupus erythematosus [**Fig. 6**E], psoriasis, nummular eczema, lichen sclerosis, and porphyria cutanea tarda).[15–19,47–49]

Interestingly, common dermatologic conditions in Africa, which typically are not associated with HIV, such as vitiligo, postinflammatory hyperpigmentation (**Fig. 7**), oculocutaneous albinism, acne vulgaris, and dermatosis papulosa nigra, were also among the most commonly in HIV patients of this Botswana dermatology cohort diagnosed. This is potentially reflective of the high penetrance of antiretroviral (ARV) therapy in the country. Botswana has one of the most successful HIV programs in the world, with widespread free access to HIV diagnosis and treatment, with an estimated 83% of the HIV population on ARV treatment.[45] Studies have shown that since the advent of ARVs, which can allow HIV to be well controlled with viral suppression, chronic noncommunicable diseases are becoming more prevalent. Instead of needing specialized care primarily for HIV-associated opportunistic diseases, the authors' HIV patients may be starting to present with the more epidemiologically common dermatologic conditions within their overall population.[50,51] Thus, it is of utmost importance that physicians caring for HIV patients have basic knowledge to diagnose and treat both HIV-associated and generally common dermatologic conditions. HIV/acquired immunodeficiency syndrome is known to confer a 90% lifetime risk of developing a skin condition; however, baseline screening questions and treatment guidelines for common dermatologic conditions are lacking for this population.[48,52] In

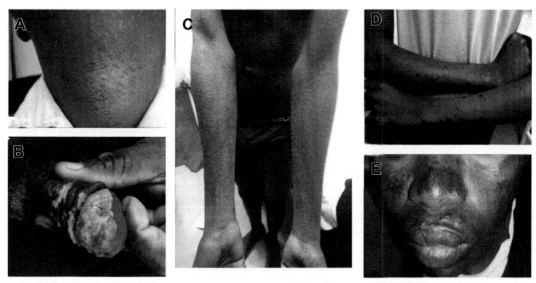

Fig. 6. (*A*) Widespread hyperpigmented flat-topped papules on the neck in an HIV-positive child with flat warts. (*B*) Moist verrucous plaques of chronic verrucous herpes simplex virus on the penis in an HIV-positive patient. (*C*) Diffuse eczematous eruption in an HIV-positive patient. (*D*) Scattered hyperpigmented excoriated papules on the extremities in an HIV-positive patient with papular pruritic eruption of HIV. (*E*) Photodistributed annular violaceous patches and thin plaques with erythematous borders in an HIV-positive patient with discoid lupus erythematosus.

high-prevalence HIV populations like Botswana, dermatologic guidelines should be developed and incorporated into standard HIV care, as has been done with conditions, such as TB or diabetes.

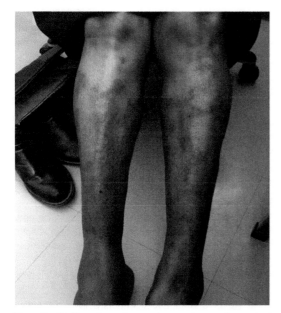

Fig. 7. Scattered polymorphous hyperpigmented patches on the legs in an HIV-positive patient with postinflammatory hyperpigmentation after resolution of a previous inflammatory eruption in the same area.

The Role of Primary Care in Dermatology

A majority (62.6%) of visits in the authors' study were follow-up visits; this reflects the difficulty the dermatology clinic at Princess Marina Hospital faces in discharging patients back to primary care to allow adequate room for new patient visits. When specialists are scarce, subspecialty consultations should aim at diagnosing conditions and outlining a treatment plan that can then be carried out by a local primary care provider. Acne, eczema, and vitiligo are common examples of conditions that can be diagnosed and managed outside of a tertiary dermatology clinic. Potential reasons that patients return to the authors' dermatology clinic after discharge include time pressure and patient volume in primary care clinic, cultural norms of referring patients to specialty clinic, providers not reading prior dermatology notes, providers discomfort in managing dermatology conditions, and patient preference for expert opinions. Because the current number of dermatologists is insufficient to meet the demand in Botswana and many developing countries, general practitioners must have access to training that will allow them to manage common skin conditions, practice stricter triage of patients into dermatology clinics, and educate patients on appropriate use of specialty care.

Increasing the ability of local providers to care for dermatologic conditions is an essential component of improving dermatologic care in Botswana. Potential interventions include organizing formal workshops and educational programs in which local dermatologists teach primary providers, expanding and formalizing existing telemedicine consultation networks, and ensuring that students and trainees receive adequate education on common dermatologic conditions in both HIV-positive and HIV-negative patients.[26,53] Previous studies from Mali and rural areas in Mexico have reported improved patient outcomes after 1-day training courses on skin diseases, indicating the benefit that even short, focused training sessions can have on dermatology care in a primary care setting.[11,54]

Limitations

The authors' study is limited by its retrospective nature, which may be subject to incomplete data and reporting bias. The authors cannot confirm the accuracy of the clinical diagnoses that were made without histologic confirmation, which is an inevitable reality in resource-limited settings. Additionally, the authors were unable to distinguish repeat visits by the same patient, so patients who presented to clinic multiple times within the study time frame could be counted multiple times. This gives an accurate picture of clinic visits but limits the ability to determine disease prevalence within the study population and can lead to an over-representation of conditions that need frequent follow-up or for conditions in patients that lived closer to clinic and were able to come for frequent follow-up. Data were collected from only 1 clinical location in the capital city, which may not be generalizable to all populations in Botswana. Future studies that collect data from a larger population, over a longer duration of time, and analyze unique patient visits and unique diagnoses would provide a more complete picture of the epidemiology of skin diseases in Botswana.

SUMMARY

This study is the first step in understanding the epidemiology of dermatologic disease in Botswana and can be used to guide future development of dermatology as a specialty in the country. The authors highlight how the high HIV prevalence in Botswana has had an impact on the overall patterns of dermatologic disease at their tertiary referral clinic. Approximately one-third of new and follow-up patients were HIV positive and commonly presented with a variety of inflammatory, infectious, vascular, neoplastic, and other pigmentary disorders. KS was the condition diagnosed most frequently in the HIV-positive

population and the most common overall histopathologic diagnosis in the cohort. Given the shortage of dermatology specialists in Botswana, the present study should be used as a guide to prioritize the allocation of resources for management of dermatologic conditions that are common in this population, such as eczematous eruptions; viral and fungal infections; skin neoplasms, including KS; vascular disorders; disorders of pigmentation; and disorders resulting from mechanical/physical injury. Medical education curriculums and continuing medical education workshops for general practitioners and HIV specialists should target these common skin conditions in order to improve access and alleviate the burden on tertiary hospitals.

ACKNOWLEDGMENTS

The authors are grateful for the support of the American Academy of Dermatology Resident International Grant and the Kramer Family Development Fund, which have supported dermatology care in Botswana for more than 10 years.

REFERENCES

1. James SL, Abate D, Abate KH, et al. Global, regional, and national incidence, prevalence, and years lived with disability for 354 diseases and injuries for 195 countries and territories, 1990–2017: a systematic analysis for the Global Burden of Disease Study 2017. Lancet 2018;392(10159): 1789–858.

2. Tuckman A. The potential psychological impact of skin conditions. Dermatol Ther 2017;7(Suppl 1): 53–7.

3. Dalgard FJ, Bewley A, Evers AW, et al. Stigmatisation and body image impairment in dermatological patients: protocol for an observational multicentre study in 16 European countries. BMJ Open 2018; 8(12):e024877.

4. Mastrolonardo M, Diaferio A, Vendemiale G, et al. Seborrhoeic dermatitis in the elderly: inferences on the possible role of disability and loss of self-sufficiency. Acta Derm Venereol 2004;84(4):285–7.

5. Picardi A, Mazzotti E, Pasquini P. Prevalence and correlates of suicidal ideation among patients with skin disease. J Am Acad Dermatol 2006;54(3): 420–6.

6. Wootton CI, Bell S, Philavanh A, et al. Assessing skin disease and associated health-related quality of life in a rural Lao community. BMC Dermatol 2018;18(1):11.

7. Kimball AB, Resneck JS Jr. The US dermatology workforce: a specialty remains in shortage. J Am Acad Dermatol 2008 Nov;59(5):741–5.

8. Resneck JS, Kimball AB. Who else is providing care in dermatology practices? Trends in the use of nonphysician clinicians. J Am Acad Dermatol 2008;58(2):211–6.

9. Yusuf SM, Musa BM, Nashabaru I, et al. Health seeking behaviour of patients with skin disorders in Kano, Nigeria. J Turk Acad Dermatol 2014;8.

10. AlGhamdi KM, Khurrum H, Asiri Y. The welcoming attitude of dermatologists towards complementary and alternative medicine despite their lack of knowledge and training. Saudi Pharm J 2017; 25(6):838-843.

11. Mahé A, Faye O, N'Diaye HT, et al. Integration of basic dermatological care into primary health care services in Mali. Bull World Health Organ 2005; 83(12):935–41.

12. Hay R, Estrada R, Grossmann H. Managing skin disease in resource-poor environments - the role of community-oriented training and control programs. Int J Dermatol 2011;50(5):558–63.

13. Statistics Botswana |. Available at: http://www. statsbots.org.bw/. Accessed May 10, 2020.

14. Botswana. Available at: https://www.unaids.org/en/ keywords/botswana. Accessed May 10, 2020.

15. The Electives Network. Princess Marina Hospital. Available at: https://www.electives.net/hospital/73/ preview. Accessed May 10, 2020.

16. Botswana Population (2020) - Worldometer. Available at: https://www.worldometers.info/world-population/ botswana-population/. Accessed May 10, 2020.

17. Botswana Overview. Available at: https://www.worldbank. org/en/country/botswana/overview. Accessed May 10, 2020.

18. WHO | Integrating noncommunicable disease services into primary health care, Botswana. Available at: http://www9.who.int/bulletin/volumes/97/2/18-221424/ en/. Accessed May 10, 2020.

19. Tapera R, Moseki S, January J. The status of health promotion in Botswana. J Public Health Afr 2018; 9(1):699.

20. Dlova NC, Chateau A, Khoza N, et al. Prevalence of skin diseases treated at public referral hospitals in KwaZulu-Natal, South Africa. Br J Dermatol 2018; 178(1):e1–2.

21. Dlova NC, Mankahla A, Madala N, et al. The spectrum of skin diseases in a black population in Durban, KwaZulu-Natal, South Africa. Int J Dermatol 2015;54(3):279–85.

22. Rosenbaum BE, Klein R, Hagan PG, et al. Dermatology in Ghana: a retrospective review of skin disease at the Korle Bu Teaching Hospital Dermatology Clinic. Pan Afr Med J 2017;26:125.

23. Parthasaradhi A, Al Gufai AF. Pattern of skin disease in Hail region of Saudi Arabia. J Dermatol Dermatol Surg 2017;21(2):62–5.

24. Bissek A-CZ-K, Tabah EN, Kouotou E, et al. The spectrum of skin diseases in a rural setting in Cameroon (sub-Saharan Africa). BMC Dermatol 2012;12:7.

25. Yahya H. Change in pattern of skin disease in Kaduna, north-central Nigeria. Int J Dermatol 2007; 46(9):936–43.

26. WHO | Epidemiology and management of common skin diseases in children in developing countries. Available at: https://www.who.int/maternal_child_ adolescent/documents/fch_cah_05_12/en/. Accessed May 10, 2020. 27.

27. Accorsi S, Barnabas GA, Farese P, et al. Skin disorders and disease profile of poverty: analysis of medical records in Tigray, northern Ethiopia, 2005-2007. Trans R Soc Trop Med Hyg 2009;103(5): 469–75.

28. De Luca DA, Maianski Z, Averbukh M. A study of skin disease spectrum occurring in Angola phototype V-VI population in Luanda. Int J Dermatol 2018;57(7):849–55.

29. Gibbs S. Skin disease and socioeconomic conditions in rural Africa: Tanzania. Int J Dermatol 1996; 35(9):633–9.

30. Marks M, Sammut T, Cabral MG, et al. The prevalence of scabies, pyoderma and other communicable dermatoses in the Bijagos Archipelago, Guinea-Bissau. PLoS Negl Trop Dis 2019;13(11). https://doi.org/10.1371/journal.pntd.0007820.

31. Hogewoning A, Amoah A, Bavinck JNB, et al. Skin diseases among schoolchildren in Ghana, Gabon, and Rwanda. Int J Dermatol 2013;52(5): 589–600.

32. Onyekonwu CL, Ojinmah UR, Ozoh GaO, et al. Epidemiology of skin diseases in University of Nigeria Teaching Hospital, Ituku-Ozalla, Enugu State. Niger J Med 2016;25(3):272–81.

33. York K, Dlova NC, Wright CY, et al. Primary cutaneous malignancies in the Northern Cape Province of South Africa: A retrospective histopathological review. S Afr Med J 2016;107(1):83–8.

34. Beltraminelli H, Kiprono S, Zuriel D, et al. Dermatopathology in sub-Saharan Africa: a systematic 5-year analysis of all histopathological diagnoses from the Regional Dermatology Training Centre (RDTC) in Moshi, Tanzania. J Eur Acad Dermatol Venereol 2015;29(7):1370–5.

35. Nthumba PM, Cavadas PC, Landin L. Primary cutaneous malignancies in sub-Saharan Africa. Ann Plast Surg 2011;66(3):313–20.

36. Adhikari RC, Shah M, Jha AK. Histopathological spectrum of skin diseases in a tertiary skin health and referral centre. J Pathol Nepal 2019;9(1): 1434–40.

37. Santos M, Vilasboas V, Mendes L, et al. Lymphangiectatic Kaposi's sarcoma in a patient with AIDS. An Bras Dermatol 2013;88(2):276.

38. Liakos D, Sofianos C, Sooka HN, et al. Vascularised free lymph node transfer - a procedure for

secondary lymphoedema management in South Africa. S Afr J Surg 2019;57(1):60–3.

39. Kamdem F, Mapoure Y, Hamadou B, et al. Prevalence and risk factors of peripheral artery disease in black Africans with HIV infection: a cross-sectional hospital-based study. Vasc Health Risk Manag 2018;14:401–8.

40. Kayıran O, De La Cruz C, Tane K, et al. Lymphedema: From diagnosis to treatment. Turk J Surg 2017;33(2):51–7.

41. Cloete N. Chronic venous disorders. S Afr Med J 2014;104(2):147.

42. Chike-Obi CJ, Cole PD, Brisset AE. Keloids: pathogenesis, clinical features and management. Semin Plast Surg 2009;23(3):178.

43. Gupta S, Khan W, Krishna A. Pattern of skin diseases and common drugs prescribed in dermatology OPD of an Indian tertiary care hospital. Int J Basic Clin Pharmacol 2016;6(1):203–7.

44. Pathak AK, Kumar S, Kumar M, et al. Study of drug utilization pattern for skin diseases in dermatology OPD of an indian tertiary care hospital - a prescription survey. J Clin Diagn Res 2016;10(2):FC01–5.

45. Botswana. Available at: https://www.unaids.org/en/regionscountries/countries/botswana. Accessed May 10, 2020.

46. BWA_2018_countryreport.pdf. Available at: https://www.unaids.org/sites/default/files/country/documents/BWA_2018_countryreport.pdf. Accessed May 10, 2020.

47. Motswaledi HM. Common dermatological conditions in the HIV patient. South Afr Fam Pract 2019;61(1). https://doi.org/10.4102/safp.v61i1.5049.

48. Hu J, McKoy K, Papier A, et al. Dermatology and HIV/AIDS in Africa. J Glob Infect Dis 2011;3(3):275.

49. Shittu RO, Odeigah LO, Mahmoud AO, et al. Dermatology Quality of Life Impairments among Newly Diagnosed HIV/AIDS-Infected Patients in the University of Ilorin Teaching Hospital (Uith), Ilorin, Nigeria. J Int Assoc Provid AIDS Care 2013. https://doi.org/10.1177/2325957413488207.

50. Kansiime S, Mwesigire D, Mugerwa H. Prevalence of non-communicable diseases among HIV positive patients on antiretroviral therapy at joint clinical research centre, Lubowa, Uganda. PLoS One 2019;14(8). https://doi.org/10.1371/journal.pone.0221022.

51. Achwoka D, Waruru A, Chen T-H, et al. Noncommunicable disease burden among HIV patients in care: a national retrospective longitudinal analysis of HIV-treatment outcomes in Kenya, 2003-2013. BMC Public Health 2019;19. https://doi.org/10.1186/s12889-019-6716-2.

52. Paul S, Evans R, Maurer T, et al. Treatment of Dermatological Conditions Associated with HIV/AIDS: The Scarcity of Guidance on a Global Scale. AIDS Res Treat 2016;2016. https://doi.org/10.1155/2016/3272483.

53. Murase JE. Understanding the importance of dermatology training in undergraduate medical education. - PubMed - NCBI. Available at: https://www.ncbi.nlm.nih.gov/pubmed/26114062. Accessed May 10, 2020.

54. Estrada R, Chavez-Lopez G, Estrada-Chavez G, et al. Specialized dermatological care for marginalized populations and education at the primary care level: Is community dermatology a feasible proposal? Int J Dermatol 2012;51:1345–50.

Yaws, *Haemophilus ducreyi*, and Other Bacterial Causes of Cutaneous Ulcer Disease in the South Pacific Islands

Camila G-Beiras, PhD[a],*, Maria Ubals, MD[a,b], Marc Corbacho-Monné, MD[a], Martí Vall-Mayans, MD[a,b], Oriol Mitjà, PhD[a,b]

KEYWORDS

- Cutaneous ulcers • Yaws • Haemophilus ducreyi • South Pacific islands
- Neglected tropical diseases

KEY POINTS

- Cutaneous ulcers are a painful and debilitating condition endemic to poor and remote regions, like the South Pacific islands and West Africa, with poor sanitation and limited health care access.
- Cutaneous ulcers in the South Pacific are caused by a range of bacterial pathogens that are not easily distinguished on clinical diagnosis.
- Syndromic management for CUD should be updated and adapted to the availability of drugs and diagnostic tools in each setting.
- New information on the causative agents of cutaneous ulcers calls for new terminology, new diagnostic tools, and more effective antimicrobial therapies.

INTRODUCTION TO CUTANEOUS ULCERS

Cutaneous ulcers (CU) are endemic in poor and remote populations, mainly in the South Pacific islands (SPIs) and West Africa. Known predisposing factors are poor access to clean water and sanitation and limited access to the health system. In the SPIs, studies from Papua New Guinea (PNG), Vanuatu, and Solomon Islands report that CUs are highly prevalent among the young population (5–15 years).[1] These lesions cause stigma among endemic populations, and children affected with CUs usually do not attend school until the ulcer is resolved. Furthermore, CU can develop into permanently impairing conditions. The terms used to refer to ulcerative conditions in the tropics are not common or not well defined in the literature, and multiple communicable and noncommunicable diseases can cause ulcers in tropical countries.

Genital ulcer disease is a syndrome characterized by ulcerating lesions on the genital area. In general usage, the term refers to genital ulcerations from a sexually transmitted infection, which is the most common etiology; however, nonsexually acquired illnesses, including infectious (bacterial skin infections and fungi) or noninfectious etiologies (fixed drug eruption, Behçet disease, and sexual trauma), can present with similar ulcers.[2] Therefore, the authors suggest that the term, *cutaneous ulcer disease (CUD)*, could be

---

[a] Fight AIDS and Infectious Diseases Foundation, Badalona, Catalonia, Spain; [b] Hospital Universitari Germans Trias i Pujol, Barcelona, Catalonia, Spain
* Corresponding author.
E-mail address: cgonzalez@flsida.org
Twitter: @camilagbeiras (C.G.-B.)

Dermatol Clin 39 (2021) 15–22
https://doi.org/10.1016/j.det.2020.08.002
0733-8635/21/© 2020 Elsevier Inc. All rights reserved.

used to describe nonvenereal skin ulcers sharing some clinical and epidemiologic characteristics. This term would need to be redefined as empirical data become available.

CU can be noninfectious, such as vascular or neuropathic ulcer or, more commonly, infectious. Infectious nonbacterial CU include cutaneous leishmaniasis, caused by several *Leishmania* species, and some, rather rare, viral or fungal infections. Bacterial CU can be caused by yaws (caused by *Treponema pallidum pertenue*), *Haemophilus ducreyi*, and polymicrobial ulcers (also called tropical or phagedenic ulcers), which often refers to ulcers that are allegedly caused by *Fusobacterium*, *Bacillus fusiformis*, *T vincentii*, and *Bacteroides*.[3] Finally, Buruli ulcer is caused by *Mycobacterium ulcerans*, which is rarely found in the SPIs.[4]

For the purpose of this review, the term CUD is used to refer to ulcers caused mainly by bacterial infections, which are endemic in the SPIs, namely (1) yaws, (2) *H ducreyi*, and (3) polymicrobial ulcers. CUD is transmitted mostly by direct skin-to-skin, nonsexual contact and typically present as single or multiple skin lesions with epidermal loss due to the sloughing of inflamed necrotic tissue. Children wearing scanty clothing, overcrowding in huts at night, and lack of soap and water for bathing all are thought to favor transmission.[1] The most common locations are the legs and arms; it is frequently chronic (ie, >2 weeks duration) and often painful.

CUTANEOUS ULCER DISEASE IN THE SOUTH PACIFIC ISLANDS
Yaws

Yaws, caused by *T pallidum subsp Pertenue*, is included in the list of neglected tropical diseases (NTDs) since 2007.[5] A systematic review published in 2015 reported that 84% of CUD caused by yaws were from 3 countries—PNG, Solomon Islands, and Ghana.[6] Yaws occurs primarily in children under 15 years of age[7] in rural, humid, tropical regions, causing painful ulcers in the skin. It causes a chronic relapsing treponematosis, characterized by a primary and secondary stage, that causes highly infectious lesions (ulcers and papilloma) (**Fig. 1**A, B), and a tertiary noncontagious stage that, if left untreated, can lead to destructive lesions of the bone[6] (**Fig. 1**C, D).

Primary and secondary lesions may heal spontaneously, and the infection can become latent at any time,[8] with only serologic evidence of infection, and relapses can occur for up to 5 years to 10 years, evolving into the tertiary stage in approximately 10% of cases.[5]

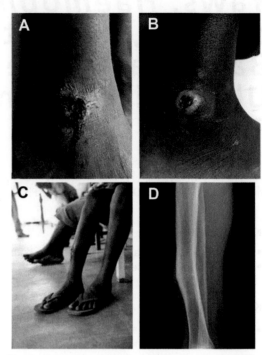

Fig. 1. Examples of classical cases of yaws including (*A*) yaws ulcer, (*B*) yaws papilloma, (*C*) yaws tertiary-stage lesion, and (*D*) yaws tertiary-stage radiograph showing typical sabre shin.

Haemophilus ducreyi

Traditionally, and due to lack of molecular confirmation tests in rural areas, all CUD have been clinically diagnosed as yaws, but recent studies conducted in the South Pacific have identified *H ducreyi* as an important etiologic agent of CUD in rural environments of tropical countries.[7,9–14]

The role of *H ducreyi* in the causation of nongenital skin ulcers first was reported in 1989 in a 22-year-old Danish traveler returning from Fiji with a chronic foot ulcer secondary to a swimming injury.[15] Subsequently, 7 other cases were reported, all of them presenting with leg ulcers after travels to the Pacific Islands countries and territories.[16–19]

The real extent of *H ducreyi* skin ulcers was demonstrated in several surveys conducted in yaws-endemic areas of PNG,[11] Vanuatu,[7] Solomon Islands,[12] and Ghana.[14] Mitjà and colleagues[11] conducted a prospective cohort study in PNG in 2013 and found that 54 (60%) of 90 participants with skin ulcers were positive for *H ducreyi* on PCR, whereas 31 (34%) cases had *T pallidum subsp Pertenue* DNA; 12 (13%) cases had mixed *H ducreyi* and *T pallidum subsp Pertenue*. Schoolchildren were most affected (mean 10 years of age; range 2–40 years). Marks and colleagues[12] undertook cluster-based surveys in the Solomon

Islands in 2013. *H ducreyi* was detected in 13 (32%) of 41 children found with exudative ulcers and serologic findings were consistent with yaws in 12 (29%) cases. In Vanuatu, Chi and colleagues,[20] examined 155 children with moist ulcers; *H ducreyi* DNA was detected in 60 (39%) cases, whereas *T pallidum subsp Pertenue* DNA was detected in 24 (15%) cases. In 2017, a study reported similar results in PNG—out of 273 ulcers, 13.5% were positive for *T pallidum subsp Pertenue*, 47.9% for *H ducreyi*, and 28.8% had negative PCR for both. The remaining 9.9% had mixed infection with yaws and *H ducreyi*.[9]

In parallel, a study in Ghana[13] reported that *H ducreyi* DNA was identified in 49 (27%) of 179 skin ulcers on real-time PCR. Ghinai and colleagues[14] undertook a cross-sectional study of ulcerative lesions in children of 2 districts who had received MDA with azithromycin for trachoma, 8 lesions (9%) of 90 participants with moist CU enrolled were positive for *H ducreyi*.

H ducreyi CUs often occur in yaws endemic areas.[7,10–12,14] Both, H ducreyi and T pallidum subs pertenue CU present with similar phenotypical appearance and demographic characteristics[7] (**Fig. 2**). Lesions caused by *H ducreyi* are extremely difficult to distinguish clinically from yaws lesions and may be found in patients who either are seropositive or seronegative for yaws. A study comparing clinical characteristics of CUs found that both yaws and *H ducreyi* ulcer characteristics were very similar, although it reported that yaws ulcers where significantly more likely to affect boys and men and present as deep round ulcers with a an elevated border compared *H ducreyi*.[9] *H ducreyi* DNA has been found alongside *T pallidum subsp Pertenue* in yaws-like lesions in several studies, and 3% to 13% of children with *H ducreyi*–positive ulcers either were coinfected with *T pallidum subsp Pertenue* or had serologic evidence of past infection with yaws.[9,11]

Experts agree that clinical distinction among these two CU is unreliable except in classical cases, which are uncommon[7] (see **Fig. 2**). The World Health Organization (WHO) recommends that health workers consult the WHO's yaws recognition booklet for further information on identification of yaws ulcers[21] or the skin NTDs pictorial guideline.[22] This guide was designed for the use by frontline health workers without specialist knowledge and comes with a phone app that helps identifying all types of CU among other NTDs (Skin NTDs App).

H ducreyi is a fastidious organism, which makes culture particularly challenging, and there are no

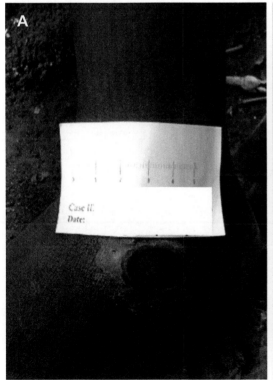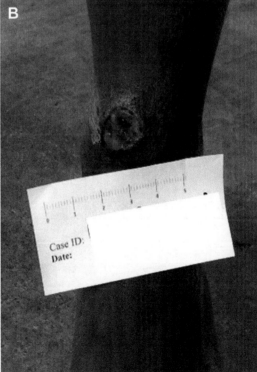

Fig. 2. Examples of cutaneous ulcers caused by (*A*) *H ducreyi* and (*B*) *T p pertenue*, which share characteristics.

point of care tests available; therefore, diagnosis is confirmed through PCR. Due to its high proportion among CUD, H ducreyi should be highly suspected upon negative rapid plasma reagin (RPR) serology in yaws endemic areas.

Polymicrobial Ulcers

The term, *tropical ulcer*, or phagedenic ulcer, often has been used in tropical medicine as a general term to define all CU identified in tropical areas. Nowadays, this term sometimes is used to describe a group of polymicrobial ulcers caused by anaerobes and gram-positive cocci. *Fusobacterium*, *Bacillus fusiformis*, and *T vincentii*, together with *Bacteroides*, are the main bacteria isolated in those ulcers.[3] The authors believe that the term, tropical ulcer, is vague and unspecific and propose that the term, *polymicrobial ulcers*, be used to describe this group.

These ulcers easily are differentiated from the rest of CUD, described previously. They commonly present with more severe manifestations: large, deep, exudative ulcers with foul-smelling thick purulent slough that tends to bleed easily[23] (**Fig. 3**).

Polymicrobial ulcers are treated mainly based on clinical diagnosis, because no testing for this type of ulcer is available in most endemic settings.

NEWLY RECOGNIZED POLYMICROBIAL PATHOGENS

A recent shotgun metagenomic study has shed new light on new potential causative agents of CU, showing significant abundance of several ulcer-associated bacteria, such as *Streptococcus dysgalactiae*, *Arcanobacterium haemolyticum*, and *Corynebacterium diptheriae*.[24] These ulcers shared clinical and epidemiologic characteristics with yaws and H ducreyi–caused CUD but tested negative in culture and polymerase chain reaction (PCR) analysis; therefore, clinical diagnosis is challenging.[9] Whether each of these pathogens is a causative agent or a colonizer is still to be confirmed.

TREATMENT AND MANAGEMENT OF CUTANEOUS ULCER DISEASE IN THE FIELD

CUD in most resource-poor countries normally is treated empirically with penicillin derivatives.

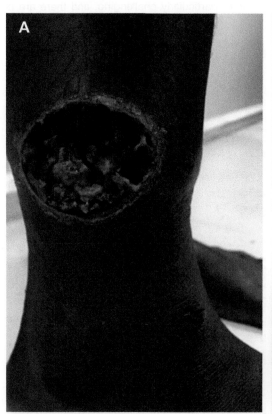 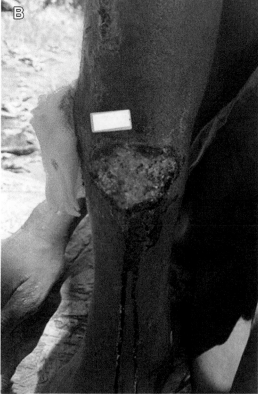

Fig. 3. *A)* and *B)* suspected polymicrobial ulcers with negative serology and negative PCR results for T pallidum subs pertenue and H dureyi.

Long-acting benzathine penicillin G, given intramuscularly is one of the recommended treatments. 1.2 MU (0.6 MU for children under 12 years), is used when yaws is suspected. The recent discovery that 1 single oral dose of azithromycin is as effective as intramuscular penicillin to treat yaws has promoted modification of first-line treatment to azithromycin because of ease of administration.[25] Since then, the WHO recommends azithromycin, 30 mg/kg (to a maximum of 2 g for adults) orally, when yaws is confirmed serologically.[26] Ulcers with a negative syphilis (yaws) serology typically are treated with penicillin derivatives. A study confirming the efficacy of single-dose azithromycin to treat *H ducreyi*, also reported that that greater than 70% of PCR negative ulcers healed fully after treatment with azithromycin, and that greater than 85% improved at 2 weeks' follow-up. These ulcers had clinical manifestation similar to *H ducreyi* and yaws ulcers.[9]

The authors propose a flowchart for syndromic management in combination with WHO recommendations to treat CUD based on clinical manifestations and the diagnostic and therapeutic options available (**Fig. 4**).

1. Clinical diagnosis: following clinical characteristics alone, azithromycin is recommended when a yaws-like ulcer is suspected. Because *H ducreyi* and yaws share common clinical characteristics, is likely that *H ducreyi* ulcers will be treated when looking for yaws-like ulcers. At 2 weeks of no clinical resolution, penicillin is recommended as second-line treatment, particularly in areas where macrolide resistance is suspected. When a polymicrobial ulcer is suspected, anaerobicides, such as metronidazole alone or in combination with gram-positive drugs, should be considered.
2. Serologic confirmation: with positive RPR serology (≥1:8) or with a Dual Path Platform Dual Path Platform (Chembio DPP®) syphilis rapid test, positive for nontreponemal antibodies, the same treatment of clinically suspected yaws is recommended. Upon a negative serology, if a polymicrobial ulcer is suspected, the authors recommend anaerobicides; with yaws-like clinical characteristics, azithromycin still is recommended because *H ducreyi* is the most likely causative agent. Amoxicillin commonly is found in rural settings and also can be used.
3. PCR test: with a confirmation of *T pallidum subsp Pertenue*, azithromycin as first-line treatment and penicillin as second-line treatment are recommended. If *H ducreyi* PCR is

confirmed, azithromycin still is the recommended drug. Upon negative PCR results, the authors recommend that the clinical characteristics of the ulcer are considered; if polymicrobial infection is suspected, treat with anaerobicides; otherwise, penicillin derivates are recommended.

Antiseptic wound cleaning, dressing, gauzing, and promotion of hygiene practices are recommended in all cases.[22]

Mass Drug Administration and Eradication Campaigns

The WHO Morges strategy observes the use of mass azithromycin treatment of affected communities.[26] Studies in the SPIs and Ghana have reported a steep decrease in the prevalence of yaws and *H ducreyi* CU lesions with the use of mass treatment strategies,[10,27] as well as the prevalence of latent yaws.[8,28] Mitjà and colleagues reported a re-emergence of yaws 3.5 years after 1 round of mass azithromycin to the community of Lihir Island, PNG, followed by biannual targeted case treatment.[29] The increase of active yaws started 2 years after the initial intervention. Given the reported high effectiveness of single-dose azithromycin for treating latent yaws, it is suspected that the relapse could have occurred from untreated latent yaws and, to a lesser extent, to reintroduction from other untreated communities, rather than from azithromycin treatment failure. In this article, Mitjà stresses the need to target broader geographic regions, especially in communities with intensive migration, and the need for close surveillance after mass drug interventions to monitor resurgence and detect drug resistance.

One of the main concerns regarding the use of mass drug strategies is the emergence of *T pallidum subsp Pertenue* macrolide–resistant strains in the communities. Mitjà and colleagues[29] reported the emergence of 5 azithromycin-resistant *T pallidum subsp Pertenue* cases within 1 village at 32 months and 42 months after mass drug administration followed by targeted case treatment every 6 months. A subsequent study, using bacterial whole-genome sequencing of the resistant samples, concluded that given the genomic and epidemiologic linkage of resistant cases and the rarity of resistance alleles in the general population, it is likely that azithromycin resistance evolved in 1 person and was later disseminated to other contacts.[30]

The data published after mass administration with azithromycin in PNG suggested a weaker effect on the reduction of the proportion of *H ducreyi* CU. These results are puzzling considering that the

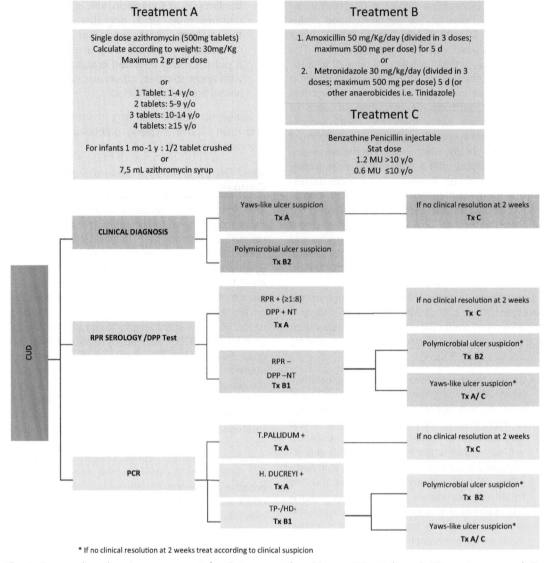

Fig. 4. Proposed syndromic management for Cutaneous Ulcer Disease. HD, *H ducreyi*; NT, nontreponemal; Tx, treatment.

high efficacy of single-dose azithromycin on *H ducreyi* CU recently was reported.[9] There are several possible explanations. First, *H ducreyi* strains that cause skin lesions in children probably are more infectious than *T pallidum subsp Pertenue*, and chancroid appears more easily transmitted than syphilis. Second, natural infection with *H ducreyi* does not appear to induce any immunity to subsequent infection, unlike the transient immunity that occurs after treponemal infection.[31] Third, the colonization of nongenital skin in asymptomatic villagers and the possible carriage of bacteria by flies may contribute to the continued presence of infection after preventative interventions.[1] Fourth, a recent selective pressure

analysis of *H ducreyi* cutaneous ulcers before and after mass treatment using single nucleotide polymorphisms concluded that in contrast to *T pallidum subsp Pertenue*, which showed a strain diversity reduction after MDA, *H ducreyi* strain composition is not affected by antibiotic pressure, which is consistent with environmental reservoirs of *H ducreyi*.[32]

This data suggest that environmental reservoirs must be addressed to achieve elimination of *H ducreyi*. The challenge posed by the ubiquity of *H ducreyi* may be addressed through repeated mass treatment with azithromycin,[1] which may confer a prophylactic effect to the population for long enough to clear the asymptomatic reservoirs.[33]

Current Efforts and Ongoing Studies

The WHO is promoting yaws eradication campaigns throughout endemic regions of West Africa and the South Pacific. The authors' team is planning further studies in the etiology and in the syndromic management for CUD to correctly manage all possible causes of CU, and the authors are working on the assessment of multiple rounds of mass drug administration for the elimination of yaws. Further projects to validate molecular testing of ulcers in the field also are under way.

FINAL REMARKS

The authors consider CUD a neglected disease of special interest, so new strategies to control it should be explored. This review should be considered a mere proposal to discuss terminology and a syndromic approach to CUD, which must be combined according to clinical and diagnostic resources on site. Validation studies of this and other syndromic approaches are needed.

DISCLOSURE

Maria Ubals holds a Río Ortega Scholarship for PhD students.

REFERENCES

1. Houinei W, Godornes C, August K, et al. Haemophilus ducreyi DNA is detectable on the skin of asymptomatic children, flies and fomites in villages of Papua New Guinea. PLoS Negl Trop Dis 2017;11(5):e0004958.
2. World Health Organization. Guidelines for the management of sexually transmitted infections 2003. Available at: http://applications.emro.who.int/aiecf/web79.pdf. Accessed May 18, 2020.
3. Adriaans B, Hay R, Drsasar B, et al. The infectious aetiology of tropical ulcer—a study of the role of anaerobic bacteria. Br J Dermatol 1987;116(1):31–7.
4. Omansen TF, Erbowor-Becksen A, Yotsu R, et al. Global epidemiology of Buruli ulcer, 2010-2017, and analysis of 2014 WHO programmatic targets. Emerg Infect Dis 2019;25(12):2183–90.
5. Mitjà O, Asiedu K, Mabey D. Yaws. Lancet 2013;381(9868):763–73.
6. Mitjà O, Marks M, Konan DJP, et al. Global epidemiology of yaws: a systematic review. Lancet Glob Health 2015;3:324–31.
7. Fegan D, Glennon MJ, Kool J, et al. Tropical leg ulcers in children: more than yaws. Trop Doct 2015. https://doi.org/10.1177/0049475515599326.
8. Mitjà O, González-Beiras C, Godornes C, et al. Effectiveness of single-dose azithromycin to treat latent yaws: a longitudinal comparative cohort study. Lancet Glob Health 2017;5(12):e1268–74.
9. González-Beiras C, Kapa A, Vall-Mayans M, et al. Single-dose azithromycin for the treatment of haemophilus ducreyi skin ulcers in papua new guinea. Clin Infect Dis 2017;65(12):2085–90.
10. Mitjà O, Houinei W, Moses P, et al. Mass treatment with single-dose azithromycin for yaws. N Engl J Med 2015;372:703–10.
11. Mitjà O, Lukehart SA, Pokowas G, et al. Haemophilus ducreyi as a cause of skin ulcers in children from a yaws-endemic area of Papua New Guinea: a prospective cohort study. Lancet 2014;14:1–7.
12. Marks M, Chi K, Vahi V, et al. Haemophilus ducreyi associated with skin ulcers among children, Solomon Islands. Emerg Infect Dis 2014;20(10):1705–7.
13. González-beiras C, Marks M, Chen CY, et al. Epidemiology of haemophilus ducreyi infections. Emerg Infect Dis 2016;22(1):1–8.
14. Ghinai R, El-Duah P, Chi K-H, et al. A cross-sectional study of 'yaws' in districts of ghana which have previously undertaken azithromycin mass drug administration for trachoma control. PLoS Negl Trop Dis 2015;9(1):e0003496.
15. Marckmann P, Højbjerg T, von Eyben FE, et al. Imported pedal chancroid: case report. Genitourin Med 1989;65(2):126–7.
16. Ussher JE, Wilson E, Campanella S, et al. Haemophilus ducreyi causing chronic skin ulceration in children visiting Samoa. Clin Infect Dis 2007;44(10):e85–7.
17. McBride WJH, Hannah RCS, Le Cornec GM, et al. Cutaneous chancroid in a visitor from Vanuatu. Australas J Dermatol 2008;49(2):98–9.
18. Humphrey S, Romney MAS. Haemophilus ducreyi leg ulceration in a 5-year-old boy. J Am Acad Dermatol 2007;56(2):AB121.
19. Peel TN, Bhatti D, De Boer JC, et al. Chronic cutaneous ulcers secondary to Haemophilus ducreyi infection. Med J Aust 2010;192(6):348–50.
20. Chi K-H, Danavall D, Taleo F, et al. Molecular differentiation of treponema pallidum subspecies in skin ulceration clinically suspected as yaws in vanuatu using real-time multiplex PCR and serological methods. Am J Trop Med Hyg 2015;92(1):134–8.
21. World Health Organisation. Yaws: recognition booklet for communities. 2012. reprinted with changes, 2014. WHO library cataloguing-in-Publication data. book ISBN 978 92 4 150409 6 Available at: https://www.who.int/yaws/resources/9789241504096/en/ Accessed May 2 2020.
22. World Health Organization. Recognizing neglected tropical diseases through Changes on the skin. 2018. ISBN: 978-92-4-151353-1 Available at: https://www.who.int/neglected_diseases/resources/9789241513531/en/. Accessed May 17, 2020.

23. Adriaans B. Royal society of tropical medicine and hygiene joint meeting with the royal society of medicine sections of dermatology and tropical medicine 19 march 1987: Tropical ulcer—a reappraisal based on recent work. Trans R Soc Trop Med Hyg 1988; 82(2):185–9.

24. Noguera-Julian M, González-Beiras C, Parera M, et al. Etiological characterization of the cutaneous ulcer syndrome in papua new guinea using shotgun metagenomics. Clin Infect Dis 2019;68(3):482–9.

25. Mitjà O, Hays R, Ipai A, et al. Single-dose azithromycin versus benzathine benzylpenicillin for treatment of yaws in children in Papua New Guinea: an open-label , non-inferiority , randomised trial. Lancet 2012;379(9813):342–7.

26. World Health Organization. Eradication of yaws—the Morges strategy. Wkly Epidemiol Rec 2012;87: 189–94.

27. Aziz Abdulai A, Agana-Nsiire P, Biney F, et al. Community-based mass treatment with azithromycin for the elimination of yaws in Ghana—results of a pilot study. PLoS Negl Trop Dis 2018;(3). https://doi.org/10.1371/journal.pntd.0006303.

28. Marks M, Sokana O, Nachamkin E, et al. Prevalence of active and latent yaws in the solomon islands 18 months after azithromycin mass drug administration for trachoma. PLoS Negl Trop Dis 2016;10(8):1–9.

29. Mitjà O, Godornes C, Houinei W, et al. Re-emergence of yaws after single mass azithromycin treatment followed by targeted treatment: a longitudinal study. Lancet 2018;0(0):1–9.

30. Beale MA, Noguera-Julian M, Godornes C, et al. A genomic epidemiology investigation of yaws re-emergence and bacterial drug resistance selection. medRxiv 2020. https://doi.org/10.1101/2019.12.31.19016220.

31. Spinola SM, Bong CTH, Faber AL, et al. Differences in host susceptibility to disease progression in the human challenge model of Haemophilus ducreyi infection. Infect Immun 2003;71(11):6658–63.

32. Grant JC, González-Beiras C, Amick KM, et al. Multiple Class i and Class II haemophilus ducreyi strains cause cutaneous ulcers in children on an endemic Island. Clin Infect Dis 2018;67(11):1729–35.

33. Thornton a C, O'Mara EM, Sorensen SJ, et al. Prevention of experimental Haemophilus ducreyi infection: a randomized, controlled clinical trial. J Infect Dis 1998;177(6):1608–13.

Telemedicine/Technology

Telemedicine and Community Health Projects in Asia

Anil Kumar Jha, MD, FRCP[a],[*],[1], Erika Sawka, BS[b],[1], Bhagirath Tiwari, MScIT[a], Huiting Dong, MD, DMSc[c], Choon Chiat Oh, MD, MRCP, M.Sc[d], Seyedali Ghaemi, MD[c], Xuejiao Zhang, MD[e], Adarsh Kumar Jha, MBBS[a]

KEYWORDS

- Telemedicine • Teledermatology • Dermatology • Store and forward • Live streaming
- Information and communication technology

KEY POINTS

- With widespread advances in technology, telemedicine initiatives have launched in several Asian countries with differing levels of economic development.
- Several of these initiatives have been successful in providing affordable, accessible, and innovative health care and education.
- Common challenges in implementing a telemedicine program have been reflected in the literature, such as difficulty maintaining financial sustainability, technological infrastructure, and integration into government and nongovernment health care systems.
- The authors highlight an example program in Nepal, the Community Health Education Services by Telehealth, which attributes its success to local collaboration, financial sustainability, and integrated community development.
- Further evaluation of the effectiveness of these programs is required in order to provide recommendations for optimal telemedicine implementation.

INTRODUCTION

Remote regions around the world face several barriers in providing accessible, cost-effective, and high-quality health care services. These barriers include socioeconomic constraint, complex geographic locations, poor infrastructure, and lack of trained health care professionals in the region. Hospitals and specialists are often concentrated in urban areas, requiring patients to travel long distances to receive care. Telemedicine, or the delivery of health care services through information and communication technologies (ICT), has the potential to reduce disparities in health care, improve health outcomes, and provide education to health care providers.[1]

Telemedicine is gaining popularity in Asia and has been used to increase access to health care providers in rural communities. Recent advances in technology, such as the use of smartphones, improved Internet infrastructure, digitalized information, and electronic medical records, have made telemedicine possible.[2] eHealth is an

Conflict-of-interest statement: No conflicts of interest to disclose.
[a] DI Skin Health and Referral Center P Ltd, Maharajgunj, Kathmandu 44600, Nepal; [b] Oregon Health & Science University, Center for Health and Healing Building, 3303 S Bond Ave #1 Mail Code 16d, Portland, OR 97239, USA; [c] Department of Dermatology, The First Affiliated Hospital, Zhengzhou University, 1 Eastern Jianshe Road, Erqi District, Zhengzhou, China; [d] Singapore General Hospital, 20 College Road, Academia, Singapore 169856; [e] Eastern District Branch, Beijing Emergency Medical Center, No. 103 Qian Men Xi Da Jie, Beijing, China
[1] These authors contributed equally.
* Corresponding author.
E-mail address: dranilkjha@hotmail.com

Dermatol Clin 39 (2021) 23–32
https://doi.org/10.1016/j.det.2020.08.003

umbrella term that encompasses ICT used for health services, whereas mHealth is specifically defined as the utilization of mobile and wireless technologies. In low- and middle-income regions, mobile phone use has grown rapidly in recent years, which has now made access to telemedicine feasible for previously unreachable parts of the world.[3]

There are several methods of providing telemedicine consultation services. Interactions may be coordinated between providers, or directly between a provider and a patient. Communication may be real-time (synchronous) audio and visual conferencing or store-and-forward (asynchronous) consultations. Telemedicine typically requires an easy-to-use interface, a communication system, technology infrastructure, and trained users.[4]

The authors' aim is to highlight numerous telemedicine and teledermatology initiatives in Asian countries. Telemedicine can be leveraged in a variety of ways, and the type of telemedicine tools used depends heavily on the needs and resources of a population. Thus, the authors organized this review by gross national income (GNI) per capita in US dollars, a World Bank classification, in order to present various telemedicine initiatives in the context of the country's economic status. During the 2020 fiscal year, low-income economies are defined as a GNI per capita less than $1025, lower-middle-income economies between $1026 and $3995, upper-middle-income economies between $3996 and $12,375, and high-income economies greater than $12,376.[5] Although GNI per capita has limitations and may not completely capture the level of development in a country, it is a practical and useful indicator of local economies and frequently correlates with nonmonetary quality-of-life measures.[6]

In addition to reviewing several initiatives, the implementation and outcomes of a successful program in Nepal are described in detail. By reviewing the goals, operations, implementation, challenges, and achievements of these programs, the authors hope to assist in the development of telemedicine in other regions struggling to meet the health care needs in both high- and low-resource settings.

HIGH-INCOME ECONOMIES
Japan

To help mitigate the rising total cost of health care, regional disparities in health care resources, and the effects of an aging population, Japan's Ministry of Finance has significantly invested in the development of telemedicine. Several services connect providers to specialists in fields, such as dermatology, radiology, and pathology, and their cost-effectiveness was evaluated in a recent systematic review. Akiyama and Yoo[7] reported that teledermatology and teleradiology systems demonstrated promising results in economic efficiency. For example, a 2-year trial of a live interactive teledermatology system reportedly saved $360 per consultation per week primarily based on reduced travel costs and time. Another study similarly concluded that these teledermatology consultations are more economical than conventional face-to-face visits.[8]

Telemedicine has also been used to host an international research and education consortium based out of Kyushu University Hospital in Fukuoka, Japan. The consortium, the Asia-Pacific Advanced Network, connected more than 50 medical institutions in 13 countries using a digital video transport system (DVTS) with a network bandwidth of 30 Mbps per channel. Several telecommunication sessions and conferences using this technology were hosted from 2003 to 2007 as well. Most participants were satisfied with the quality of the system.[9] DVTS may be a simple, cost-effective tool with the potential to connect a broad audience of health care workers for continuing education even when they are separated by location.

Singapore

As one of the most advanced economies in Asia with high capacity for ICT, Singapore has had several teledermatology initiatives studied. A Web-based teledermatology system was evaluated among patients with nonurgent skin conditions in a nursing home. A personal electronic health record management system was used to send store-and-forward consults to dermatologists who responded with a diagnostic report and treatment plan. A survey of nurses and consulting dermatologists demonstrated satisfaction with the system in its ability to provide convenient and effective care; however, it was thought that some skin conditions may require face-to-face consultation in order to provide an accurate diagnosis. The study suggested dermatologic care would be best provided with a combination of teledermatology and traditional in person health care delivery.[10]

Seghers and colleagues[11] conducted a small prospective study at the Institute of Mental Health in Singapore to compare teledermatology via real-time videoconferencing with face-to-face consultation in a group of institutionalized psychiatric patients with chronic skin diseases. They concluded that teledermatology was as effective as face-to-face consultation in regard to diagnostic accuracy and management outcomes based on a high level of agreement between the types of consultations. In addition, the utilization of teledermatology in this group demonstrated the possibility of reduced total turnaround time, reduced need for resources to coordinate external medical appointments and provide transportation, and increased patient comfort. This study highlights the potential benefits of teledermatology in mental health institutions.

UPPER-MIDDLE-INCOME ECONOMIES
China

As China is the country with the world's largest population, a substantial portion of the Chinese population lives in rural areas, and there are significant regional disparities in medical resources. Telemedicine has been used in China to alleviate geographic limitations and provide specialized medical services.[12] One of the 3 major telemedicine networks, the People's Liberation Army, was established in the early 1990s and has expanded to include more than 200 military and civil hospitals and 300 specialists. The goal of this nationwide military health information network, which is funded by the Chinese government, is to provide specialty care to both members of the military and civilians in urban and rural areas.[13] In 2001, a retrospective study found that the largest portion of teleconsultations was for orthopedic complaints with only 1.8% for dermatologic concerns.[14] With the many advances in teledermatology to date, it is likely that this number has grown. Challenges this program has faced included lower than expected overall network utilization, inadequate telephone data transfer rates in rural areas, and 63% satisfaction with teleconsultation sessions.[14]

The National Telemedicine Center of China, formerly the Henan Province Telemedicine Center of China, is a cross-regional system established more than 20 years ago at the First Affiliated Hospital of Zhengzhou University.[12,15,16] Initially, the center referred a small number of patients to larger hospitals using real-time teleconsultation. In the early 2000s, the center expanded to provide referral services to various hospitals and performed several hundred patient care consultations.[15,16] By 2018, the system had grown in the number of administrative staff and researchers and increased its referring hospitals to include 147 referring hospitals across China[16,17] as well as one in Africa (Huiting Dong, personal communication, November 2018). The number of teleconsultations has rapidly grown from 2322 cases in 2014 to 14,445 cases in 2018,[16,17] and 22,248 cases in 2019 (Huiting Dong and Chuan Jiang, personal communication, May 2020).

The rapidly expanding use of smartphones in China provides an opportunity to develop mHealth initiatives in order to improve access to health care services for underserved populations. A recent systematic review of more than 300 mHealth interventions in China found that most interventions were conducted in urban areas through mobile applications, such as WeChat. In some specialties, more than 95% of interventions were conducted in cities where specialists are concentrated. In addition, cardiology, endocrinology, behavioral health, and oncology were the most common specialty services provided, with few specialty services focused on dermatology. Future mHealth initiatives have the opportunity to alleviate the maldistribution of specialty services in urban and rural areas as well as target underrepresented specialties like dermatology.[18]

Iran

Although physician visits are generally inexpensive in Iran, Web-based consultation services have become a popular method of seeking medical advice. A prospective study evaluated one of these "ask-the-doctor" services that was launched in 2009.[19,20] Patients fill out an online form with the option to include a photograph, and a consultation is sent to volunteer physicians, free of charge. Although some "ask-the-doctor" services are public forums, this Web site is private. The most frequently asked questions were regarding sexual health, women's health, mental health, gastrointestinal issues, and cosmetic concerns. About half of the submissions were fully answered, and about a third were partly answered or led to additional in-person referrals. Because patients were responsible for providing their own clinical descriptions, difficulties with definitive diagnosis and treatment often arose, in addition to ethical implications. However, the platform did provide a consult service for patients who may be reluctant to speak openly to their physician about sensitive health-related topics, and about half of users found the advice they received effective.[19]

LOWER-MIDDLE-INCOME ECONOMIES
Vietnam

Vietnam has faced challenges with limited resources in remote areas, high prevalence of communicable diseases, and lack of affordable health care. With widespread use of mobile phones, access to high-speed Internet among most of its citizens, and existing service coverage in remote areas, mHealth is emerging as a method to allow high-quality delivery of health care. Lam and colleagues[21] recently identified 20 mHealth initiatives in Vietnam, with the majority hoping to improve health in marginalized and hard-to-reach populations. Services provided include general health education through the use of SMS, a free counseling hotline, and support systems for health practitioners. According to the study, major barriers of continuing to provide mHealth services include lack of financial sustainability owing to dependence on foreign funding, poor technological infrastructure, difficulty communicating between the various Vietnamese dialects, and lack of supportive government policies.

Vietnam's National HIV Program, initially funded by international donors, has been successful in vastly improving treatment delivery and training community health care workers in human immunodeficiency virus (HIV) care. However, medical expertise remained concentrated in a few specialized institutions, and trainees were required to travel long distances for mentorship. In 2014, the Vietnam HIV Telehealth Program was formed to help overcome these barriers by providing training and expert consultation using the videoconferencing platform, Zoom. Over a period of 4 years, the program grew to encompass 17 public institutions and 700 clinical sites across almost every province in Vietnam. An evaluation of the program revealed high levels of satisfaction and improved competence of HIV clinical management among health care workers. The program made note of the importance of aligning with the national government's health strategies and plans, pursuing financial sustainability, adapting delivery of evidence-based health care services, and providing training and capacity building to local staff. Ultimately, the telehealth program has helped ease the HIV program's transition from international donor funding to domestic support, enabling more long-term sustainability.[22]

Bangladesh

The Ministry of Health and Family Welfare in Bangladesh provides a telemedicine service between specialized, district, and subdistrict hospitals. Provider-to-provider consultations are made through video conferencing platforms, such as Skype.[23] A mobile health service has also been developed, in which patients can call for free medical advice from physicians working in government hospitals.[24] The purpose of this program is to provide immediate medical advice to patients of all socioeconomic groups, particularly in rural areas.

A pilot project with Grameenphone by Telenor, the leading telecommunications service provider in Bangladesh, was initiated in 2012 in collaboration with the Telemedicine Working Group of Bangladesh.[25] The intent was to provide dermatologic care to patients in rural areas using mobile Internet connection. Patients connect directly with physicians over video conferencing to receive quick, affordable care. Reports in 2014 demonstrated success with about 4500 consultations performed in 3 pilot sites. The program has added several telemedicine centers in rural sites and has plans to expand its health services.[26]

Hossain and colleagues[27] explored the factors involved in a successful eHealth program in Bangladesh. A survey of residents in a rural district found that social reference, advertisement, attitude toward the system, access to a cellphone, and perceived system effectiveness were the most influential variables in accepting eHealth tools. The study provided an understanding of the values of potential eHealth users and recommendations for successful program implementation.

India

As the second most populated country in the world, India has been using eHealth to reach its more vulnerable citizens for several years. The Apollo Telemedicine Networking Foundation is a nonprofit organization established in 1999 by Apollo Hospitals, a private hospital group in India. The purpose of the organization is to offer a secure and confidential telemedicine platform to connect rural medical centers with Apollo hospitals. The Indian Space Research Organization (ISRO) has helped with the technological infrastructure by providing fiberoptic cables, adequate bandwidth, satellite-based communication, and mobile telemedicine units.[28] Now, as one of Asia's largest health care providers and multispecialty telemedicine networks, the program has expanded to include more than 50 hospitals and 4000 consultants across 50 specialties in several Asian and African countries.[29]

In 2008, the World Health Partners' (WHP) Sky Program set up telemedicine hubs in rural areas in India. "SkyHealth" clinics are franchises run by local entrepreneurs that provide audiovisual communication between patients in rural villages and urban physicians.[30] The network also includes more than 1000 local rural providers, central medical facilities that house consulting physicians, clinics for surgical and inpatient care, diagnostic facilities, and pharmacies.[31] Funding includes the WHP, investments from local entrepreneurs, and the Bill and Melinda Gates Foundation. Although an incentive-based entrepreneurial model is an innovative telemedicine concept, Mohanan and colleagues[32] evaluated quality of care and clinical outcomes of 2 common childhood conditions (diarrhea and pneumonia) and did not find evidence of significant improvement. The overall effectiveness of the program has thus been questioned.[33]

There are several additional telemedicine programs in India.[2] Under the Ministry of Health and Family Welfare and the Department of Information Technology, a National Telemedicine Portal has been created for education and eHealth delivery. The National eHealth Authority, a separate program, aims to provide cost-effective and secure health services. Furthermore, about 500 Village Resource Centers developed by the ISRO have been formed across the country. They function as learning centers and telemedicine connectivity hubs as well as provide local information on the weather, water management, and fisheries.

Pakistan

More than 65% of the population in Pakistan lives in rural areas and faces geographic challenges when accessing affordable and quality health care.[34] To combat the shortage of health care services in these areas, Telenor, a large telecommunications company servicing countries across Asia, launched a telemedicine service in 2008 following their success in Bangladesh. For their more than 26 million mobile phone subscribers, they offer 24/7 access to medical advice from experienced physicians. Basic health information and assessment of health complaints are available in various languages.[13]

Mongolia

Clinics in remote and medically underserved areas in Mongolia have been using a mobile phone platform for store-and-forward teledermatology consultations. In 2013, Byamba and colleagues[35] performed a randomized controlled trial at 20 different clinic sites to evaluate the usefulness of an electronic medical record system and mobile phone software that provided image-taking techniques, health care questionnaires, and decision-making trees. Providers used these resources to gain relevant clinical information to include in their consultation to a dermatologist. When compared with a control group that did not receive training or this software, they found that there was a 75% reduction in the number of referrals to tertiary-care centers in the intervention group. This study shows that mHealth services have the potential to reduce patient travel times and financial burdens.

Cambodia

An mHealth initiative has been established in Cambodia in order to link female entertainment workers, a population that is at risk of poor sexual and reproductive health owing to direct or indirect sex work, to health services. A recent randomized controlled trial evaluated the effectiveness of this mHealth intervention in improving health outcomes in this population.[36] Thus far, results have demonstrated participants' interest in gynecologic issues, cervical cancer, and breast cancer over HIV and family planning. It has been suggested that incorporating participatory methodologies, tailoring the platform at the individual level, and building trust were aspects of the mHealth program that are likely to make it successful.[37]

LOW-INCOME ECONOMIES
Nepal

The Nepal Research and Education Network in partnership with Nepal Wireless Networking Project, a local Internet provider, has been delivering telemedicine services since 2006.[38] The network collaborates with Kathmandu Model Hospital as well as several others in the region. Weekly education sessions, workshops, and conferences are hosted over video using the network's high-bandwidth capabilities.[39] The network supports existing telemedicine initiatives, including the Communication Health Education Services by Telehealth, which will be described in more detail in later discussion.[38]

The Department of Health Services of Nepal launched a telemedicine program in 2009 out of Patan Hospital. Services included live video conferencing for consultations, an online portal with store-and-forward technology, and a medical advice hotline called "Hello Swasthya." They have serviced at least 25 districts.[38] According to recent reports, the program was discontinued for several years; however, the government is funding a revival of its telemedicine services in a few remote hospitals.[40]

Afghanistan, Tajikistan (Low Income); Kyrgyz Republic, Pakistan (Lower-Middle Income)

In 2013, the Central Asia Health Systems Strengthening Project was initiated in collaboration with the Aga Khan Foundation and the Government of Canada. The objective was to provide telemedicine services to communities in rural and isolated regions of Afghanistan, Kyrgyz Republic, Pakistan, and Tajikistan, which comprise a mix of low and lower-middle economic development levels. The network uses ICT to link patients with providers at government and nongovernment institutions through a 2-tier hub-and-spoke model. The program delivers specialty health care services to rural areas through live and store-and-forward teleconsultations. In addition, eLearning services are provided for continuous medical, nursing, and professional education. From 2013 to 2014, the program was successful in providing more than 6000 consultations and developing more than 50 eLearning modules for more than 2000 beneficiaries. This program has actively adapted in order to combat various challenges, including using fiberoptic lines and backup connectivity methods, delivering periodic technical training for health care workers, charging subsidized fees to beneficiaries to create a sustainable financial model, and hiring regional coordinators to alleviate communication and language barriers.[41]

IN DEPTH: TELEDERMATOLOGY AND COMMUNITY HEALTH PROGRAM IN NEPAL
Background

This section provides a detailed overview of the implementation and achievements of a teledermatology initiative in a low-resource setting. The Community Health Education Services by Telehealth, or C.H.E.S.T., is a nongovernment organization established in 2009 whose mission is to provide telemedicine services and vocational training to Nepalese citizens who live in remote areas without access to health care.[42] With an emergence of widespread smartphone use, C.H.E.S.T. sought to use ICT to improve the quality of life of rural villagers through health and education services. The organization is based out of the DI Skin Health and Referral Center (DISHARC) in Kathmandu, Nepal and is funded by the hospital.[43] The program was launched with the support of visiting professor, Dr Gunter Burg, Strategic Partners for Nepal (STRAPAL),[44] Swisscontact,[45] and prominent ICT activist, Mahabir Pun. Major aims are to improve overall quality of life of communities by connecting them to urban resources, including health care and education, to develop various employment and life skills.

Project Locations

C.H.E.S.T. Nepal selected 3 pilot villages (Gerkhutar, Babhangama, and Mudikuwa) to operate its services based on geographic location and low socioeconomic condition of the local community (**Fig. 1**). Villages were selected from each of the remote geographic regions of Nepal (**Fig. 2**A),

including mountains, hills, and plains, which also lacked basic government health care facilities.

Project Framework and Technical Infrastructure

With this program, patients receive free live video dermatology consultations without having to travel to specialists in urban areas. When C.H.E.S.T. arrives to a new village, a consultation center is established with equipment for audio and video communication (**Fig. 2**C). Local nonmedical volunteers are trained to manage the technical equipment and oversee consultations. The technical infrastructure comprises an optical fiber cable with dedicated 8-Mbps per second intranet connection to allow the capacity for live video streaming. A separate camera is provided to allow a mechanism for store-and-forward telemedicine. The secure intranet is used whenever possible; however, if the connection fails, WhatsApp, a mobile messaging application, can be used as an additional back up. The technical infrastructure is illustrated in **Fig. 3**.

Services Offered

C.H.E.S.T. provides telehealth services for dermatology and internal medicine in rural and remote areas of Nepal through live and/or store-and-forward teleconferencing (**Fig. 2**D, F). Communities are provided with support to build a self-sustainable telehealth and training program under their ownership to ensure sustainability. C.H.E.S.T. builds capacity through offering classes and training for the community members in ICT using the same infrastructure. Additional skill development, counseling, and training are offered in appropriate areas dictated per the needs of and resources available in the local community, such as teacher training in English language, various computer skills, and agriculture/horticulture development. This education provides the basis for building rural community development (**Fig. 2**B, E).

Project Achievements

The program currently provides weekly teledermatology services with more than 2000 patients consulted to date. C.H.E.S.T. has secured reduced-cost medications to treat skin disease in these communities. More than 20 free health check-up camps have been organized in these areas, providing a variety of health care services to more than 3000 patients. More than five hundred villagers have received computer training to improve their understanding of and ability to use ICT. Agriculture experts have provided advice for improved growing of organic vegetables and

Project Locations

Locations	Connectivity
Mudikuwa, Parbat (West Nepal)	Subisu
Gerkhutar, Nuwakot (Central Nepal)	Subisu
Babhangama, Janakpur (East Nepal)	Subisu
DISHARC premises, Central Station	Subisu

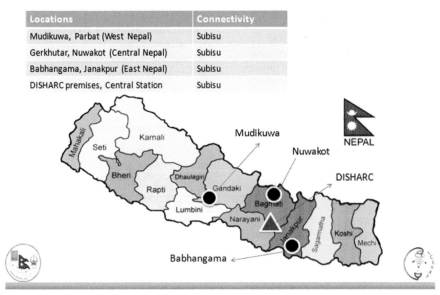

Fig. 1. C.H.E.S.T. operates out of DISHARC hospital in Kathmandu and provides telemedicine infrastructure and services in the villages of Mudikuwa, Gerkhutar, and Babhangama.

food grains within participating villages. With the support of STRAPAL, a new community building was constructed in Gerkhutar after the earthquake damage in April 2015.

A unique feature of C.H.E.S.T. is that it is run by the community. It acts as a link between a community center and DISHARC, in contrast to other telemedicine projects, which typically network between rural hospitals and city hospital. In order to ensure sustainability, partial funding is provided to each community initially to help establish the consultation center. Revenue to sustain the program is then

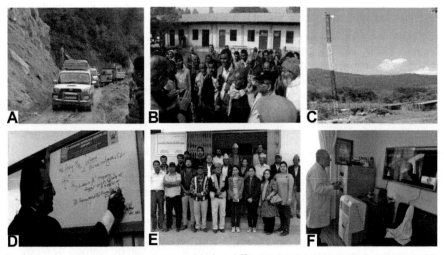

Fig. 2. Telehealth and tele-awareness services provided at different C.H.E.S.T. community centers in Nepal: (A) the road to reach Gerkhutar in the mountainous Nuwakot district is narrow and difficult, showcasing how remote C.H.E.S.T. rural village sites are; (B) community member participants in the C.H.E.S.T. initiative at the Babhangama site in the Janakpur Zone of the Terai region; (C) construction of the C.H.E.S.T. community center at Gerkhutar with assistance from STRAPAL; (D) Dr Anil K. Jha writing virtual prescriptions; (E) community member participants in front of community building in Gerkhutar; (F) Dr Anil K. Jha using video technology to perform live synchronous dermatology consults with patients at a remote C.H.E.S.T. site.

Technical Infrastructure

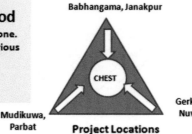

1. Real Time Streaming
- Networking made using VPN (Virtual Private Network) connected through optical fiber cable to all locations.
- It is using up to 8 Mpbs intranet speed for live video streaming.

2. Store & Forward Method
- Through e-mail & cellular smart phone.
- We are using mobile device and various mobile apps to promote mHealth initiative.

Various services provided
1. Health services
2. Skill development trainings
3. Public awareness

Babhangama, Janakpur

CHEST

Mudikuwa, Parbat

Gerkhutar, Nuwakot

Project Locations

DISHARC
DI Skin Hospital and Referral Center Pvt. Ltd

CHEST
Community Health Education Services by Tele-health

Fig. 3. The technical infrastructure of the C.H.E.S.T. program includes real-time streaming and store-and-forward methods to provide services, such as telemedicine and skill development training.

generated by minimal charges to the community members, which use the centers (specific amounts are decided by individual village communities).

Program Challenges and Opportunities

C.H.E.S.T. has successfully reached communities in remote and marginalized locations of Nepal and continues to successfully manage the program. In addition to health, this program supports social development by offering communities the chance to build concrete skills they can use to gain employment and improve their lives. In particular, the program highlights the benefits of building sustainability through telehealth centers at satellite sites connected to an informed and proactive health team. C.H.E.S.T. is committed to strengthening the program across Nepal with plans to expand regionally and incorporate additional specialty services beyond dermatology. Challenges faced include limited manpower and lack of availability of modern and innovative ICT tools in these locations, which are reducing the quality of services and sustainability of the program. Despite existing challenges, this work serves as an example for practicing community development in Nepal that other organizations can build on.[42]

LIMITATIONS

There are numerous telemedicine programs across Asia, and technology in this region is evolving rapidly. The purpose of this article is not to provide a comprehensive review of all telemedicine programs in Asia, but rather to highlight several notable initiatives and status of telemedicine adoption in different regions. This review is limited by the inability to verify the current status of programs and the lack of studies conducted to evaluate efficacy of the programs discussed.

SUMMARY

Telemedicine provides an opportunity to deliver health care services, surveillance, and education across Asia from low- to high-income economies. An overview of telemedicine initiatives provides important insights into the structure, implementation, outcomes, and challenges they have faced. There are many successful examples of telemedicine providing affordable, accessible, and innovative health care and education to remote regions in Asia. However, financial sustainability, technological infrastructure, and integration into government and nongovernment health care systems remain common challenges among these programs. Valuable lessons can be learned by studying telemedicine programs and their success in expanding regionally and integrating into the current health care landscape. Telemedicine is becoming more important in the current health care environment when face-to-face contact and travel may become limited because of unavoidable circumstances, such as the COVID-19 pandemic, environmental disasters, regional conflicts, or other security concerns. Further studies are needed to evaluate the effectiveness of several of these programs in order to provide recommendations for optimal telemedicine implementation.

ACKNOWLEDGMENTS

Community Health Education Services by Telehealth (C.H.E.S.T.) initiative received support from Dr Gunter Burg, Strategic Partners for Nepal (STRAPAL), Pierre Fabre Foundation, Swisscontact, Dr Mahabir Pun, DI Skin Health and Referral Center (DISHARC), and SUBISU Cable Net.

DISCLOSURE

The authors have nothing to disclose.

REFERENCES

1. Delaigue S, Bonnardot L, Steichen O, et al. Seven years of telemedicine in Medecins Sans Frontieres demonstrate that offering direct specialist expertise in the frontline brings clinical and educational value. J Glob Health 2018;8(2):020414.
2. Chellaiyan V, Nirupama A, Taneja N. Telemedicine in India: where do we stand? J Family Med Prim Care 2019;8(6):1872.
3. Abaza H, Marschollek M. mHealth application areas and technology combinations: a comparison of literature from high and low/middle income countries. Methods Inf Med 2017;56(7):e105–22.
4. Desai B, McKoy K, Kovarik C. Overview of international teledermatology. Pan Afr Med J 2010;6:3.
5. World Bank Country and Lending Groups. In: The World Bank. 2020. Available at: https://datahelpdesk.worldbank.org/knowledgebase/articles/906519-world-bank-country-and-lending-groups. Accessed May 14, 2020.
6. Why use GNI per capita to classify economies into income groupings? In: The World Bank. 2020. Available at: https://datahelpdesk.worldbank.org/knowledgebase/articles/378831-why-use-gni-per-capita-to-classify-economies-into. Accessed May 14, 2020.
7. Akiyama M, Yoo BK. A systematic review of the economic evaluation of telemedicine in Japan. J Prev Med Public Health 2016;49(4):183–96.
8. Dekio I, Hanada E, Chinuki Y, et al. Usefulness and economic evaluation of ADSL-based live interactive teledermatology in areas with shortage of dermatologists. Int J Dermatol 2010;49(11):1272–5.
9. Shimizu S, Nakashima N, Okamura K, et al. One hundred case studies of Asia-Pacific telemedicine using a digital video transport system over a research and education network. Telemed J E Health 2009;15(1):112–7.
10. Janardhanan L, Leow YH, Chio MTW, et al. Experience with the implementation of a web-based teledermatology system in a nursing home in Singapore. J Telemed Telecare 2008;14(8):404–9.
11. Seghers AC, Seng KH, Chio MTW, et al. A prospective study on the use of teledermatology in psychiatric patients with chronic skin diseases. Australas J Dermatol 2015;56(3):170–4.
12. Zhai Y, Gao J, Chen B, et al. Design and application of a telemedicine system jointly driven by videoconferencing and data exchange: practical experience from Henan Province, China. Telemed J E Health 2020;26(1):87–98.
13. Kimble C. Business models for E-health: evidence from ten case studies. J Org Excell 2015;34:18–30.
14. Lian P, Fu Z, Ning Y, et al. The telemedicine network of the People's Liberation Army. J Telemed Telecare 2001;7(4):187–92.
15. Miao Q, Dong H. The history of telemedicine center in our hospital. In: The 1st World Congress of Teledermatology & Annual Meeting of the Austrian Scientific Society of Telemedicine, Graz, Austria, November 9 - 11, 2006. J Dtsch Dermatol Ges 2006;4(11):999-1017.
16. Zhang X, Dong H. Rapidly growing telemedicine centre of Henan Province. In: The 1st International Conference on eHealth and Telemedicine (ICEHAT) Kathmandu 1st - 3rd November 2018. J Int Soc Telemed eHealth 2018;6(1):1-17.
17. Zhang X. Teledermatology: history and reality. In: China National Knowledge Infrastructure. 2018. Available at: https://kns.cnki.net/KCMS/detail/detail.aspx?dbcode=CMFD&dbname=CMFD201802&filename=1018107583.nh&v=MjM1MDdmWXVScUZpSG5XcnpCVkYyNkZySzRHZFRFckpFYlBJUjhlWDFMdXhlZUzdEaDFUM3FUcldNMUZyQ1VSN3E=. Accessed May 26, 2020.
18. Yang X, Kovarik CL. A systematic review of mobile health interventions in China: identifying gaps in care. J Telemed Telecare 2019. https://doi.org/10.1177/1357633X19856746.
19. Deldar K, Marouzi P, Assadi R. Teleconsultation via the web: an analysis of the type of questions that Iranian patients ask. J Telemed Telecare 2011;17(6):324–7.
20. Health for all: gateway to being healthy. Available at: https://www.telehealth.ir/. Accessed May 12, 2020.
21. Lam JA, Dang LT, Phan NT, et al. Mobile health initiatives in Vietnam: scoping study. JMIR MHealth UHealth 2018;6(4):e106.
22. Pollack TM, Thi V, Nhung T, et al. Building HIV healthcare worker capacity through telehealth in Vietnam. BMJ Glob Health 2020;5:2166.
23. Telemedicine Service. In: Government of the People's Republic of Bangladesh. Available at: https://dghs.gov.bd/index.php/en/home/84-english-root/

ehealth-eservice/490-telemedicine-service. Accessed May 12, 2020.

24. Health Service through Mobile Phone. In: Government of the People's Republic of Bangladesh. Available at: https://dghs.gov.bd/index.php/en/e-health/our-ehealth-eservices/84-english-root/ehealth-eservice/105-health-service-through-mobile-phone. Accessed May 12, 2020.

25. Connectivity to cure disease. In: Telenor Group. 2013. Available at: https://www.telenor.com/connectivity-to-cure-disease/. Accessed May 12, 2020.

26. Grameenphone Pilot teledermatology in Bangladesh. In: Grameenphone. Available at: https://www.grameenphone.com/about/corporate-information/corporate-responsibility/health. Accessed May 12, 2020.

27. Hossain N, Yokota F, Sultana N, et al. Factors influencing rural end-users' acceptance of e-health in developing countries: a study on portable health clinic in Bangladesh. Telemed J E Health 2019; 25(3):221–9.

28. Bagchi S. Telemedicine in rural India. PLoS Med 2006;3(3):297–9.

29. Ganapathy K, Ravindra A. Telemedicine in India: the Apollo story. Telemed J E Health 2009;15(6):576–85.

30. Davar M. Tele-Health delivery models in India-an analysis. In: Access Health International. 2012. Available at: https://accessh.org/reports/tele-health-delivery-models-in-india-an-analysis/. Accessed May 17, 2020.

31. Chavali A. World health partners. In: Access Health International. 2011. Available at: https://globalhealthsciences.ucsf.edu/sites/globalhealthsciences.ucsf.edu/files/pub/worldhealthpartners.pdf. Accessed May 17, 2020.

32. Mohanan M, Giardili S, Das V, et al. Évaluation d'un programme de franchises sociales et télémédecine et de la prise en charge de la diarrhée et de la pneumonie infantiles dans l'État du Bihar (Inde). Bull World Health Organ 2017;95(5):343–352E.

33. Acclaimed program Fails to Improve Health Care for Children in Rural India. In: Duke Global Health Institute. 2016. Available at: https://globalhealth.duke.edu/news/acclaimed-program-fails-improve-health-care-children-rural-india. Accessed May 13, 2020.

34. Gulzar S, Khoja S, Sajwani A. Experience of nurses with using eHealth in Gilgit-Baltistan, Pakistan: a qualitative study in primary and secondary healthcare. BMC Nurs 2013;12(1):6.

35. Byamba K, Syed-Abdul S, García-Romero M, et al. Mobile teledermatology for a prompter and more efficient dermatological care in rural Mongolia. Br J Dermatol 2015;173(1):265–7.

36. Brody C, Tuot S, Chhoun P, et al. Mobile Link – a theory-based messaging intervention for improving sexual and reproductive health of female entertainment workers in Cambodia: study protocol of a randomized controlled trial. Trial 2018;19(1):235.

37. Chhoun P, Kaplan KC, Wieten C, et al. Using participatory methods to build an mHealth intervention for female entertainment workers in Cambodia: the development of the Mobile Link project. mHealth 2019;5:24.

38. Telemedicine Services in Nepal. In: Nepal Portal. Available at: http://www.sasecrtn.edu.np/index.php/en/resources/usefulinfo/information-on-e-health-and-telemedicine/telemedicine-services-in-nepal. Accessed May 13, 2020.

39. Supporting Telemedicine. In: Nepal Research and Education Network. 2017. Available at: https://www.nren.net.np/supporting-telemedicine/. Accessed May 13, 2020.

40. Ministry of Health and Population to resume telemedicine services. In: The Kathmandu Post. 2019. Available at: https://kathmandupost.com/health/2019/09/20/government-to-resume-telemedicine-services. Accessed May 13, 2020.

41. Sajwani A, Qureshi K, Shaikh T, et al. eHealth for remote regions: findings from central Asia health systems strengthening project. Stud Health Technol Inform 2015;128–34.

42. Jha A, Gurung D. Teledermatology in Nepal: A model providing sustainable healthcare and education services helping overall community development. 2014. Available at: https://www.google.com/url?sa=t&rct=j&q=&esrc=s&source=web&cd=&cad=rja&uact=8&ved=2ahUKEwin2rSsysvrAhUpJTQIHXduAAkQFjAAegQIBhAB&url=https%3A%2F%2Filds.org%2Fdownloads.php%3Ffile2%3Dwp-content%2Fuploads%2F2018%2F04%2FCommunity_Dermatology_17.pdf&usg=AOvVaw1xRXSWGD23RFDOoqQkTjxf. Accessed May 18, 2020.

43. Legoullon P. C.H.E.S.T. Teledermatology at the service of the most isolated patients. In: Report of field survey for the e-health observatory in the southern countries of the Fondation Pierre Fabre. 2017. Available at: https://www.odess.io/files/documents/enquetes/CR_ODESS2017-CHEST_English.pdf. Accessed May 18, 2020.

44. Strategic Partnership for Nepal. In: Strapal. Available at: https://www.strapal.org/home. Accessed May 13, 2020.

45. Swisscontact – Swiss Foundation for Technical Cooperation. In: Swisscontact. 2019. Available at: https://www.swisscontact.org/en/home.html. Accessed May 13, 2020.

Utilizing Technology for Dermatology Care in Tajikistan
A Health Systems Perspective

Ali Lotfizadeh, MD, MPH[a],*, Rustam A. Sultonov, MD[b],
Ashkan Morim, MD, MPH[a,c], Sherwin Tavakol, MPH[d],
Meelod Daneshvar, MD[e], Azizullo M. Qosimov, MD[f], Toby Maurer, MD[g]

KEYWORDS

- Teledermatology • Health systems • Tajikistan • Governance • Technology • Service delivery

KEY POINTS

- In Tajikistan, where distances can be long and a large proportion of the population lives outside of major cities, teledermatology can serve as an effective method of skin care delivery.
- The authors designed a store-and-forward teledermatology program to allow dermatologists in smaller cities to consult with their most experienced colleagues in the capital city of Dushanbe on complex patient cases.
- Thus far, 228 consultations have taken place through the teledermatology platform, although several challenges to implementation exist.
- The application of a health systems framework by the World Health Organization, comprising various health systems building blocks, helped define the aims of the program and enabled putting in place needed elements to maximize program success.

INTRODUCTION

Tajikistan is a land-locked former Soviet country in Central Asia, with a population of 9 million.[1] More than 90% of the country comprises mountainous terrain[2] and a majority of the population lives in rural regions.[3] Following the collapse of the Soviet Union in 1991, Tajikistan became an independent country.[4] Although the official language is Persian, until recently, medical education was conducted almost entirely in Russian. The bulk of resources used by medical professionals also are in Russian.

Health care in Tajikistan is delivered predominantly through the public sector, constituting more than 98% of outpatient services.[5] This applies to dermatologic care as well, which is delivered through national, provincial, and city-level skin hospitals as well as city and township health facilities.[6] Patients with skin conditions are treated on outpatient and inpatient bases through dermatology services. The reason for hospitalization usually is to increase adherence with treatment regimens or to accommodate patients who have traveled long distances.

[a] PASHA, Los Angeles, CA, USA; [b] Sughd Oblast Dermatology Hospital, Khujand, Tajikistan; [c] Department of Emergency Medicine, University of California Riverside, 4445 Magnolia Avenue, Riverside, CA 92501, USA; [d] Keck School of Medicine of USC, 1975 Zonal Avenue, Los Angeles, CA 90033, USA; [e] Department of Surgery, UCSF Fresno Medical Center, 155 N. Fresno Street, Fresno, CA 93701-2302, USA; [f] Ministry of Health and Social Protection of the Population, Shevchenko Street 69, Dushanbe 734000, Tajikistan; [g] Indiana University School of Medicine, 545 Barnhill Drive, Emerson Hall 139, Indianapolis, IN 46202, USA
* Corresponding author. PO Box 64166, Los Angeles, CA 90064.
E-mail address: ali@pasha4health.org

Dermatol Clin 39 (2021) 33–41
https://doi.org/10.1016/j.det.2020.08.004

There are a total of 230 dermatologists in Tajikistan, all of whom work in the public sector.[6] Postgraduate training in dermatology involves a minimum of 1 year of dermatology internship, which is required to practice as a dermatologist. Some dermatologists, who seek academic or leadership positions, opt for an additional 2 years of clinical and/or research training. Dermatology residents are placed at the National Republic Center for Dermatology and Venereology (NRCDV), the Dushanbe City Dermatology Hospital, or the Sughd Oblast Dermatology Hospital in the northern city of Khujand.

NRCDV provides tertiary care for patients with skin conditions from all over the country. Many of the dermatologists at this center are highly respected as they collaborate with colleagues from Russia, other former Soviet countries, Western Europe, and South Asia. As a result, patients frequently self-refer to this hospital, traveling long distances to seek medical care at this center. This can be both costly and difficult for patients, however, especially in the winter months, when road and weather conditions are not optimal.

The authors' objective was to design a telemedicine program to achieve the following primary aims: (1) improve quality of care by enabling local dermatologists to consult with experts at NRCDV, (2) reduce patient self-referral to NRCDV, and (3) improve knowledge among dermatologists outside of Dushanbe and trainee dermatologists by putting in place a reliable mechanism for teledermatology consultations. These efforts are in keeping with the Ministry of Health and Social Protection's of the Population (MOHSP) goal of ensuring that all individuals receive high-quality equitable dermatologic care.

METHODS
Approach

The authors applied the World Health Organization (WHO) health systems conceptual framework to design a teledermatology program with the overarching goal of ensuring high quality, equitable, dermatologic care. This conceptual framework proposes 6 key building blocks as essential to the functioning of a health system: (1) health service delivery, (2) human resources for health, (3) health governance, (4) health information, (5) technologies and medical products, and (6) health financing (**Fig. 1**).[7]

By applying this framework, the authors were able to consider the minimum elements needed within each building block for successful implementation of the teledermatology program. The framework also enabled designing the program

in a way that would, in turn, further strengthen the various building blocks as they relate to the delivery of dermatologic care.

Details of the Teledermatology Platform and Infrastructure

This program was planned as a collaboration between PASHA, a United States nonprofit organization, and the MOHSP, with funding support from an American Academy of Dermatology Skin Care for Developing Countries grant. Local dermatologists and ministry officials provided extensive feedback on the program at all stages of implementation. One aim of this program was to enable dermatologists from smaller cities to consult with their more experienced colleagues at the NRCDV on patients with complex skin conditions. The public dermatology clinic or hospital in the cities of Kulob, Qurghonteppa, Khujand, and Vahdat (hereafter referred to referring sites) were selected as facilities that would consult with NRCDV on complex cases using teledermatology (**Fig. 2**). These 4 sites were chosen because they are among the most populous cities in Tajikistan and serve large rural populations within their vicinity. At each of the referring sites and at the NRCDV, PASHA provided and installed computers. Google Drive was used to transmit patient information. A Google account was created for each referring site as well as the NRCDV. PASHA staff, along with a local dermatologist from the NRCDV and a Tajik medical student, provided training on the use of Google Drive. The training and installation of the hardware and software occurred between January and July of 2017.

Dermatologists at referring sites were trained to use the software to consult with dermatologists at the NRCDV on cases where they felt a second opinion would improve management. For patients where a teledermatology consultation was deemed appropriate, the dermatologist at the referring site entered the patient's name, date of birth, chief complaint, history of present illness, past medical history, medications, and any relevant laboratory test results into corresponding cells of a Google Sheet. The referring physicians used their personal smartphones to take photos of skin. These photos then were transferred to the computer with a cable and subsequently uploaded into a cell in the same Google Sheet. Two dermatologists at NRCDV regularly checked the Google Drive folders, reviewed the sheets, and took turns providing a diagnosis and treatment plan, which then was implemented by the dermatologist at referring sites at patient follow-up. All providers

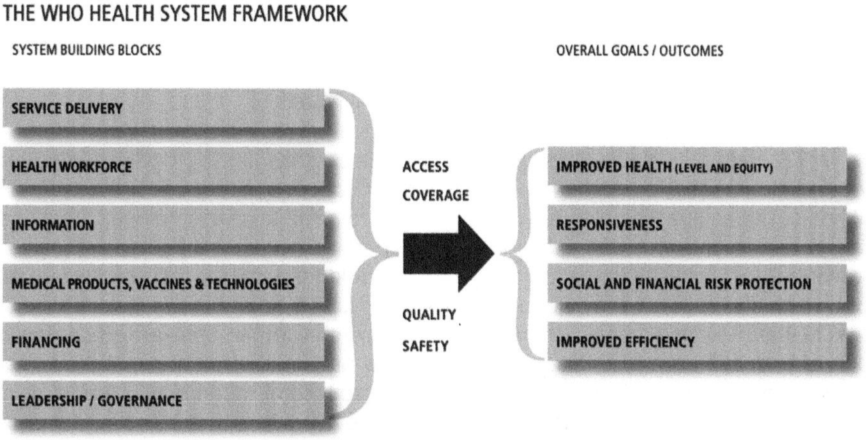

THE WHO HEALTH SYSTEM FRAMEWORK

SYSTEM BUILDING BLOCKS

OVERALL GOALS / OUTCOMES

SERVICE DELIVERY

HEALTH WORKFORCE

INFORMATION

MEDICAL PRODUCTS, VACCINES & TECHNOLOGIES

FINANCING

LEADERSHIP / GOVERNANCE

ACCESS
COVERAGE

QUALITY
SAFETY

IMPROVED HEALTH (LEVEL AND EQUITY)

RESPONSIVENESS

SOCIAL AND FINANCIAL RISK PROTECTION

IMPROVED EFFICIENCY

Fig. 1. WHO building blocks—the 6 building blocks of the WHO health systems framework work together to achieve the goal of improved health, responsiveness to patient needs, protection from financial and social risk, and increased efficiency. (*From* Everybody's Business - Strengthening health systems to improve health outcomes: WHO's framework for action. Geneva 2007.)

purchased their own data plans to connect to the Internet using USB modems.

Data from the teledermatology portal were collected and organized in Microsoft Excel. In instances where the dermatologist at NRCDV provided a diagnosis, the authors translated that diagnosis into English and classified the diagnoses into different skin disease categories according to the *International Classification of Diseases, Tenth Revision*.[8] Unstructured open-ended interviews

were conducted with individual dermatologists at NRCDV and the referring sites, along with roundtable discussions, to identify barriers to consultation and determine ways to enhance the teledermatology program.

RESULTS

A total of 228 patients have been referred through the portal thus far. Of the total referrals, 103 were

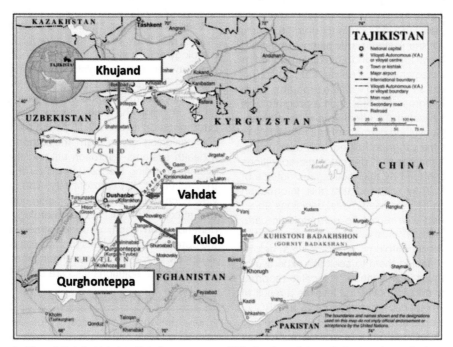

Fig. 2. The 4 cities of Kulob, Vahdat, Qurghonteppa, and Khujand used the teledermatology platform to consult with experts in Dushanbe on patients with complex skin conditions.

from the city of Khujand, 32 were from Kulob, 20 were from Qurghonteppa, and 73 were from Vahdat. Among the referred cases, 201 were reviewed by 1 of 2 consulting dermatologists at the NRCDV, who responded with a management plan in 168 of the referrals. In 122 cases, the consulting physician provided a diagnosis and, in another 12, a differential diagnosis. There were 11 instances where the consulting physician only provided a diagnosis but no treatment plan. The referring dermatologists did not provide their suspected diagnosis or treatment plan in the majority of cases. Therefore, it was difficult to determine concordance rates in diagnosis or management. In cases of the consulting physicians not providing a diagnosis or management plan, they reported that they either did not have Internet access at the time or they found it easier to call the referring physician and discuss the case by phone.

Of the 122 diagnoses provided by the consulting physician, 30 (24.6%) were dermatitis and eczema, 15 (12.3%) were disorders of skin appendages, 13 (10.6%) were papulosquamous disorders, 12 (9.8%) were infections of the skin and subcutaneous tissue, 4 (3.3%) were bullous disorders, 2 (1.6%) were urticaria and erythema, and 46 (37.7%) were other disorders of the skin and subcutaneous tissue. The 5 most common diagnoses were drug eruption (6 cases), contact dermatitis (6 cases), congenital melanocytic nevus (6 cases), dermatitis due to substances taken internally (5 cases), and onychogryphosis (5 cases) (**Table 1**).

Both consulting and referring dermatologists from each of the 4 sites participated in unstructured interviews and a roundtable discussion after program implementation. The dermatologists reported overall satisfaction with the program. There was general agreement that such a program was needed in Tajikistan and effective in enhancing patient care. Consulting dermatologists from NRCDV stated that the program helped with their understanding of the types of dermatologic conditions being encountered by their colleagues outside of the capital. They reported that this information could inform future ministry-level decisions about areas of need with regard to dermatologic care. Dermatologists from the referring sites stated that the teledermatology program was helpful because it enabled them to seek the expertise of their colleagues in Dushanbe. They also reported an increase in their knowledge level as a result of the input provided by dermatologists at NRCDV through the program. Physicians at the 4 referring sites also stated that patients who were informed that an expert from the NRCDV was providing input on their skin condition expressed satisfaction with this additional input on their care. Both consulting and referring physicians stated that the program had a positive impact on their e-health literacy.

Several challenges also were reported. Four key barriers presented by both referring and consulting dermatologists were (1) a lack of remuneration for providing teledermatology care, (2) lack of time to participate, (3) an inability to effectively incorporate teledermatology into the current workflow of daily activities as a clinician, and (4) formatting problems with the software. Referring dermatologists participating in this program reported that the process of transferring photos from their mobile device to the computer was time-consuming. They also stated that when photos were dragged into the Google Sheet, there were formatting problems with the sheet. Consulting dermatologists expressed frustration with the fact that they were unable to see the post-treatment outcomes of patients for whom they had provided a teleconsultation. Both consulting dermatologists stated that they would be more motivated to participate if they could see that their teledermatology consultations led to a positive outcome for patients.

DISCUSSION

This article describes a model of store-and-forward teledermatology between general dermatologists across different parts of Tajikistan and their counterparts at a tertiary referral skin hospital in the capital city of Dushanbe. This is the first use of teledermatology in Tajikistan and, to the best of the authors' knowledge, the first report on teledermatology across all of Central Asia. Teledermatology between dermatologists in the community and their counterparts at specialized care centers has previously been described in several other settings, including the United States and Germany, but reports on its use are limited in the literature.[9]

In designing this program, the authors employed a health systems approach utilizing the 6 health systems building blocks defined by the WHO as they relate to skin care delivery. The authors review each of these building blocks, outlining how the success of this teledermatology program depended on each, and conversely examining the potential impact of this program on each building block. Some of the challenges faced and propose potential solutions also are considered.

Health Service Delivery

A key challenge in the delivery of dermatologic care for patients residing in rural areas and smaller towns is the long distance of travel to the NRCDV in the capital city of Dushanbe, where many

Table 1
Diagnoses provided by consulting physicians according to skin disease categories from the
International Statistical Classification of Diseases and Related Health Problems

Diagnosis	Number of Cases (% of Total Cases); N = 122
Bullous disorders	4 (3.3)
Epidermolysis bullosa	2 (1.6)
Linear IgA bullous dermatosis	1 (0.8)
Pemphigus vulgaris	1 (0.8)
Dermatitis and eczema	30 (24.6)
Drug eruption	6 (4.9)
Contact dermatitis	6 (4.9)
Dermatitis due to substances taken internally[a]	5 (4.1)
Prurigo	4 (3.3)
Atopic dermatitis	3 (2.5)
Eczema	2 (1.6)
Eczema herpeticum	1 (0.8)
Posttraumatic eczema	1 (0.8)
Dyshidrosis	1 (0.8)
Lichen simplex chronicus	1 (0.8)
Disorders of skin appendages	15 (12.3)
Onychogryphosis	5 (4.1)
Alopecia	2 (1.6)
Rosacea	2 (1.6)
Sycosis	2 (1.6)
Acne vulgaris	1 (0.8)
Hirsutism	1 (0.8)
Hyperhidrosis	1 (0.8)
Onychomycosis	1 (0.8)
Infections of the skin and subcutaneous tissue	12 (9.8)
Dermatophytosis	4 (3.3)
Pyoderma	2 (1.6)
Cutaneous leishmaniasis	2 (1.6)
Demodicosis	1 (0.8)
Erysipelas	1 (0.8)
Staphylococcal scalded skin syndrome	1 (0.8)
Tinea cruris	1 (0.8)
Papulosquamous disorders	13 (10.6)
Lichen planus	4 (3.3)
Plaque psoriasis	3 (2.5)
Pityriasis rosea	2 (1.6)
Psoriasis	2 (1.6)
Palmoplantar nonpustular psoriasis	1 (0.8)
Pustular psoriasis	1 (0.8)
Urticaria and erythema	2 (1.6)
Behçet disease	1 (0.8)
Erythema multiforme	1 (0.8)
Other disorders of the skin and subcutaneous tissue	46 (37.7)
Congenital melanocytic nevus	6 (4.9)

(continued on next page)

Table 1
(continued)

Diagnosis	Number of Cases (% of Total Cases); N = 122
Pellagra	4 (3.3)
Plantar wart	3 (2.5)
Pigmented nevus	3 (2.5)
Ichthyosis	3 (2.5)
Herpes zoster	2 (1.6)
Stasis dermatitis of lower legs	2 (1.6)
Necrobiosis lipoidica	2 (1.6)
Systemic sclerosis	2 (1.6)
Venous stasis ulcer of lower extremity	2 (1.6)
Plantar hyperkeratosis	2 (1.6)
Ichthyosis vulgaris	2 (1.6)
Systemic lupus erythematosus with skin involvement	1 (0.8)
Xanthelasma	1 (0.8)
Keratoderma	1 (0.8)
Basal cell carcinoma	1 (0.8)
Nonpigmented nevus	1 (0.8)
Flat warts	1 (0.8)
Kaposi sarcoma	1 (0.8)
Lipoma	1 (0.8)
Neurofibromatoses	1 (0.8)
Palmoplantar hyperkeratosis	1 (0.8)
Lichen scleorsus	1 (0.8)
Verruca vulgaris	1 (0.8)
Oral mucosal warts	1 (0.8)
Total	122 (100)

[a] Consultant did not specify whether this was due to ingestion of food or drugs.

patients prefer to seek care because of the presence of physicians with greater expertise. One aim of this teledermatology program was to enhance health service delivery by enabling patients to seek dermatologic care at their local health facility and receive a second opinion from dermatologists in the capital when warranted, thereby obviating the need to travel long distances.

Physicians reported that time and lack of integration of teledermatology into their work flow were challenges to participating in teledermatology. Specifically, the process of transferring photos from the mobile device to the computer and formatting the images was cumbersome. To address this, the authors are in the process of moving the teledermatology platform to a software designed specifically for telemedicine and providing iPads to participating providers. With the new software and iPads, high-quality photos can be taken and uploaded onto the dermatology portal using the same device, eliminating the need for the manual transfer of photos from the mobile device to the computer. It also is expected that formatting problems will be resolved with the use of the new software. Along with these efforts, in order to increase uptake, local providers are working to raise awareness about the program within the patient community to encourage patients to seek care at the local facility in the nearest town instead of traveling to the NRCDV in Dushanbe.

Human Resources for Health

One of the 6 building blocks of the WHO health systems framework is human resources. As with all teledermatology services, this program relies on the physician workforce for its success, but it also was designed with the aim of strengthening the dermatology workforce. The teledermatology portal has the potential to increase availability of human resources for the delivery of health care services at the NRCDV by reducing the number of unnecessary in-person visits, thus freeing up time for visits with more complex patients. In the United States, the use of teledermatology at a public county hospital has had this type of positive effect, leading to increases in total volume of patients treated and reductions in patient waiting times.[10]

The portal has allowed dermatologists at referring sites to share complex cases with more experienced colleagues in Dushanbe and seek their opinion. This process also has the potential to lead to increases in the knowledge level for referring dermatologists. Although the authors did not systematically measure this, the referring dermatologists reported that the program enhanced their knowledge level. There is evidence that store-and-forward teledermatology can improve knowledge of skin disease and its treatments among primary care providers in the United States.[11] In the long term, as referring dermatologists learn the approaches used by their colleagues at the NRCDV, they may adopt similar practices and share these practices with colleagues in their region, which could, in turn, enhance the standards of dermatologic care across Tajikistan.

In addition, in the United States, there has been a move toward greater use of teledermatology in residency curricula.[12] This is a new element that the authors plan to combine with the teledermatology portal in Tajikistan. Modeled on American residency programs, the educational component will provide an opportunity for dermatology residents in Dushanbe to meet at a predefined time on a weekly basis to discuss teledermatology cases with their attending physicians at the NRCDV. The residents will review cases, come up with a differential diagnosis and treatment plan, present their assessment and plan to the attending physician, and together provide a final recommendation to referring physicians. By defining teledermatology as a component of resident education, the authors hope that the provision of teledermatology services will be integrated more effectively into the daily clinical workflow in the years to come.

Another factor related to the human resources building block is health workforce motivation. The consulting dermatologists in the authors' program reported that the inability to see final outcome of their teleconsultation made them less engaged in teledermatology. In addition to financial remuneration, intrinsic motivators, such as a desire to do good, are thought to play an important role in driving health care provider behavior.[13] With the new teledermatology software that the authors currently are introducing, the progress of a patient can be followed over time. This, in turn, may serve as an intrinsic motivator for consulting dermatologist leading them to further engage in teledermatology consultations.

Health Governance

There is consensus within the health systems literature that good governance is a key element of achieving successful health outcomes and improving access.[14] Recognizing this principle, the authors worked from the early stages of the design of this program to identify a local champion who could lead these efforts. They found this was imperative to motivating the workforce to become engaged in this program. Because the implementation of this program, the authors have also worked closely with the MOHSP to ensure there is ministry-level support for their activities. Currently, the authors are working with the MOHSP to better define the role that teledermatology can play in service delivery. This involves formally including the provision of dermatologic care through telemedicine as one of the defined responsibilities of dermatologists.

Health Information

This program has led to a collection of data and images, which provides useful information about the types of skin conditions that are deemed complex and being referred to the tertiary center for further evaluation. Although this information does not supplant epidemiologic surveys or disease registries, it has helped local providers gain a better picture of some of the complex skin conditions that may be prevalent or problematic in different regions. Information from this portal also may provide insights on the extent to which evidence-based approaches are being employed to treat skin conditions and shed light on the availability of various therapeutics in the country, because drugs that are not available presumably will not be recommended by the consulting dermatologists.

Data on the current practices and recommended therapies gleaned from the teledermatology portal currently are being used to develop clinical guidelines for the treatment of dermatologic conditions adapted to Tajikistan in collaboration with colleagues from several institutions in the United States. Additionally, according to physicians in Dushanbe, information collected from the teledermatology portal has, in part, contributed to a realization among providers that there is heterogeneity in the use of terms to describe medical or dermatologic concepts. Some physicians use Tajik-Persian terms, others use the Iranian-Persian terms, whereas others still use the Russian terms. This has prompted the Tajik Association of Dermatologists to create a dictionary to standardize the terminology.

A key part of this program has involved training of local dermatologists in the use of computer technology to enter and review patient information. Although the authors never measured this in a structural fashion, they observed that physicians using this portal are more confident and capable in using the computer software now than they were before the program was implemented. In interviews and roundtable discussions, the physicians corroborated the authors' observations by stating that the program increased their ability to use computer technology. The use of this teledermatology program also has drawn the attention of the MOHSP and providers from other specialties, who have expressed interest in developing electronic databases where they can collect information on patients with a variety of conditions. In December of 2019, PASHA provided technical assistance to endocrinologists from the MOHSP to establish an electronic database that could be piloted at 4 different endocrinology clinics across Dushanbe to collect information about patients with type 1 diabetes mellitus and type 2 diabetes mellitus. Ophthalmologists in Tajikistan also have expressed interest in using a similar approach to collect information on patients with ocular trauma.

Medical Technologies and Products

Medical products and technologies are integral elements of an effective health system. With more widespread use of telemedicine and teledermatology, computer technology both in the form of hardware and software also increasingly is recognized as a key component of this health systems building block. One way in which the authors supported this program was the provision of desktop and laptop computers at the referring centers and the NRCDV. Most of the physicians in the program used their own smartphones to take photos of the skin lesion and transferred the photos to the computer. Internet access (4G) is available across most of Tajikistan, which made it possible for referring and consulting dermatologists to use USB modems, which they personally had purchased, to access the Internet.

In conjunction with computer hardware and software, the success of this teledermatology program and dermatologic care in general is contingent on access to medicines. Progress has been made in this area in recent years. Some treatments cannot be obtained, however, within the country or at all pharmacies. One example is locally sourced Unna boots. Although the cost of production is low and the Unna boot potentially can serve as a new source of revenue for pharmacies, most pharmacies are not producing such Unna boots because the staff are not trained in their production. The authors currently are working with the Division of Pharmaceutical Services in the MOHSP to design a program that would train pharmacy staff to prepare these boots, ensuring there is enough supply to meet demands while setting prices in a way that does not make them unaffordable to patients. The authors hope that this collaboration can set the foundation for future work within this division of the MOHSP to procure other needed medications and treatments at low cost.

Health Financing

One of the major aims of this teledermatology program is to reduce the financial burden on individuals and families. As discussed previously, patients from all over Tajikistan self-refer to the NRCDV in Dushanbe to seek care from the most respected specialists in the country. Some of these individuals travel by car for 1 day to 2 days to reach the capital and incur significant transportation costs. Wages also are lost as patients and family members take time off from work. Furthermore, patients traveling from long distances often have nowhere to stay when they reach Dushanbe and, therefore, are hospitalized, which incurs additional costs to them and places a financial burden on an already stretched public health care system.[5]

Future studies examining the impact of this program would be valuable in determining if there is, in fact, a reduction in the financial burden and the extent of this reduction. Nevertheless, the current facts support the potential for reductions in expenditures. Studies from other countries also point to evidence of cost effectiveness of store-and-forward teledermatology, particularly for individuals who otherwise would have to travel long distances.[15] Recent evidence from Portugal suggests that the use of store-and-forward teledermatology in presurgical consultations for skin cancer can lead to reductions in patient out-of-pocket expenditures.[16]

Furthermore, developing a financial model for physician remuneration that would ensure sustainability of the program remains a key challenge of this program. As described previously, the absence of compensation for the time dermatologists spend on such consultations was a major barrier to participation. A clear financial scheme is needed to ensure sustainability of such a program.

SUMMARY AND FUTURE DIRECTIONS

This article highlights several lessons learned through the introduction of teledermatology in Tajikistan as well as challenges faced. Physicians on the ground report benefits from the program, including improvements in their knowledge levels, e-health literacy, and an overall ability to better care for their patients. The data suggest that there is uptake of the program by referring physicians and participation on the part of the consulting physicians. Nevertheless, challenges, such as technical difficulties with the software, may be hindering the program from achieving its full potential. There are limitations to the methodology used to evaluate the program, because baseline evaluations were not conducted nor was a control group used. Therefore, it is difficult to make definitive conclusions about the direct impact of the program on quality, outcomes, or costs. Furthermore, the diagnoses provided by the consulting physicians were not confirmed with histopathologic analysis. Therefore, it is difficult to know with certainty how accurately these diagnoses reflect the actual pathology causing skin disease in patients.

One key takeaway from the authors' experience, which they believe can be applied in other contexts, is that telehealth services and teledermatology, in particular, do not occur in isolation from the larger health system. The success of such programs and their scalability require identifying and ensuring that key health systems elements are in place. The authors found the WHO health systems conceptual framework (see **Fig. 1**) a useful metric to design a teledermatology program. Using this framework, they were able to ensure that key local health systems elements needed for the program to succeed were in place. The use of this framework also enabled designing the program with the goal of strengthening each of the health systems building blocks as they related to dermatologic care. In doing so, the authors believe that it is more feasible to achieve the long-term goal of providing high-quality equitable dermatologic care to the population. Although all health systems building blocks are relevant, the authors found that local ownership and good governance are key elements needed for the success of this program.

ACKNOWLEDGMENTS

The authors thank the American Academy of Dermatology Skin Care for Developing Countries grant, which made this work possible.

DISCLOSURE

The authors have nothing to disclose.

REFERENCES

1. Agency on Statistics under President of the Republic of Tajikistan. Available at: https://www.stat.tj/en/. Accessed March 21, 2020.
2. Country profile: Tajikistan. Washington, DC: Library of Congress - Federal Research Division; 2007.
3. World Bank Open Data. 2018. Available at: https://data.worldbank.org. Accessed March 12, 2020.
4. Rechel B, Ahmedov M, Akkazieva B, et al. Lessons from two decades of health reform in Central Asia. Health Policy Plan 2012;27(4):281–7.
5. Khodjamurodov G, Sodiqova D, Akkazieva B, et al. Tajikistan: Health System Review. Health Syst Transit 2016;18(1):1–114.
6. Health of Citiziens and Activities of Health Institutions in 2017 Dushanbe, Tajiksitan 2018.
7. Everybody's Business - Strengthening health systems to improve health outcomes: WHO's framework for action. Geneva2007.
8. International Statistical Classification of diseases and related health problems 10th Revision. Geneva: World Health Organization; 2016. Available at: https://icd.who.int/browse10/2016/en. Accessed April 6, 2020.
9. van der Heijden JP, Spuls PI, Voorbraak FP, et al. Tertiary teledermatology: a systematic review. Telemed J E Health 2010;16(1):56–62.
10. Zakaria A, Maurer T, Su G, et al. Impact of teledermatology on the accessibility and efficiency of dermatology care in an urban safety-net hospital: A pre-post analysis. J Am Acad Dermatol 2019;81(6):1446–52.
11. Mohan GC, Molina GE, Stavert R. Store and forward teledermatology improves dermatology knowledge among referring primary care providers: A survey-based cohort study. J Am Acad Dermatol 2018;79(5):960–1.
12. Wanat KA, Newman S, Finney KM, et al. Teledermatology Education: Current Use of Teledermatology in US Residency Programs. J Grad Med Educ 2016;8(2):286–7.
13. Lagarde M, Huicho L, Papanicolas I. Motivating provision of high quality care: it is not all about the money. BMJ 2019;366:l5210.
14. Witter S, Palmer N, Balabanova D, et al. Health system strengthening-Reflections on its meaning, assessment, and our state of knowledge. Int J Health Plann Manage 2019;34(4):e1980–9.
15. Snoswell C, Finnane A, Janda M, et al. Cost-effectiveness of store-and-forward teledermatology: a systematic review. JAMA Dermatol 2016;152(6):702–8.
16. de Mello-Sampayo F. Patients' out-of-pocket expenses analysis of presurgical teledermatology. Cost Eff Resour Alloc 2019;17:18.

Dermatology Education

Community Dermatology in Argentina

Isabel María del Pilar Casas, MD

KEYWORDS

- Community dermatology Argentina • Medical education • Primary care • Photoeducation
- Medical students • *Jornadas* • Health education • Workshops for children

KEY POINTS

- Around the globe there are too few dermatologists to accommodate the high demand for skin care.
- There is a huge disproportion between the need for dermatologists compared with actual activities organized by dermatologists aimed at reaching other health care workers, medical students, children, and the community as a whole.
- Education of non medical community and frontline health workers is the most effective way of producing long-term changes in skin health of large populations.
- In this article, we describe different pedagogic strategies to address each target group.

INTRODUCTION

Although medicine, as traditionally taught, has focused on the care of the individual patient, the greatest successes achieved in the improvement of human health have generally followed the implementation of programs designed to control disease in communities.[1] The expression "community dermatology" was coined by a group working in Mexico to describe a series of activities where the dermatologist's role extends beyond an individual patient to the community as a whole.[2] Medical facilities in developing countries are largely concentrated in urban areas, and most of the population has only limited access to them. There are too few dermatologists to deal with a high demand for skin care because of the high prevalence of skin diseases, and most of them are working at private practice. The aim of the Community Dermatology Argentina program is to provide accessibility through education and dermatologic expertise for rural communities that, either for geographic or socioeconomic reasons, do not have access to a specialist.

Organizations, such as the International Foundation for Dermatology[3] and the International Alliance for Global Health Dermatology[4] promote and support these types of initiatives.[5] The program started in 2009, taking as a model Professor Henning Grossman's works at the Regional Dermatology Training Center[6] in Tanzania and Professor Roberto Estrada's at Dermatología Comunitaria Mexico.[7] It consist in short periods of training of 2 working days (jornadas) held in different rural areas. They include health care (direct patient care), education (dermatology courses for health care workers), and prevention (workshops on photoprotection and prevalent skin conditions aimed at children and primary school teachers) activities. Jornadas involve volunteer fully trained dermatologists, dermatology residents, and medical students.

OBJECTIVES OF THE ARGENTINA COMMUNITY DERMATOLOGY PROGRAM

- To improve dermatologic care in rural areas through dermatology education and training of frontline health workers in the recognition of prevalent skin diseases and effective pathways of management of these conditions.
- To allow dermatologic consultation, through teledermatology or facilitated referrals, for

Comahue National University Faculty of Medicine, Comunitaria Argentina, Dermatologist at Hospital Provincial Dr. Ramón Carrillo, Av. San Martín 381, CP 8370, San Martín de los Andes, Neuquén, Patagonia Argentina
E-mail address: doctoracasas@gmail.com

Dermatol Clin 39 (2021) 43–55
https://doi.org/10.1016/j.det.2020.08.005
0733-8635/21/© 2020 Elsevier Inc. All rights reserved.

people that lack access because of geographic or socioeconomic reasons.

- To survey dermatologic pathologies in rural populations.
- To initiate activities oriented to prevent prevalent dermatoses.
- To offer medical treatment of pathologies detected.
- To analyze and share epidemiologic data obtained to stimulate research activities.

GEOPOLITICAL CONTEXT

Neuquén province is located in the southwest of Argentina, in the Cordillera de los Andes, in the border with Chile (**Fig. 1**). According to 2010 national census, Neuquén province had 551,266 inhabitants, distributed in a 94,078 km^2 area.[8] In line with global observations, few dermatologists are available in these rural areas. During the 1970s, Neuquén government established the Primary Public Health Care System, which divides the province into six health regions, each one with a medium-complexity referral hospital and many low-complexity peripheral centers. All of them are interconnected by a fluid system of patient referral from lower complexity to higher complexity level centers. The highest complexity hospital is in Neuquén capital city, located not in the geographic center of the province, but in the easternmost border (**Fig. 2**).[9] Each health division has medium- and low-complexity hospitals.[10] In the rural area surrounding low-complexity hospitals, primary attention health care posts are distributed among Mapuche communities. There is no public transportation to these communities. A monthly visit is performed by the nearest hospital staff, usually by a general physician and a dentist (**Fig. 3**).

When referral to the capital city is required, patients must travel approximately 400 km. Even at the maximum-complexity level location, accessibility to public dermatologic assistance is minimal, because there are only two dermatologists there for the entire province. Also, even though skin diseases often dominate illness patterns at the community level, there are usually many other conditions that end up taking priority over skin disease for patient referrals.[11]

Local health care workers are the key piece that allows distant rural communities to be included in the health system. They belong to Mapuche communities, and most of the time they are chosen by their own members. They receive continuous training to perform as primary-level health care givers (they deliver the medicines ordered by the doctor, help in understanding medical

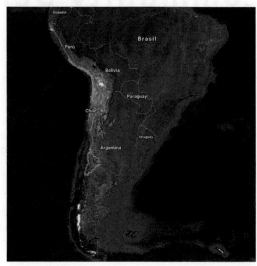

Fig. 1. Geographic location of Neuquén Province at the southwest of Argentina, close to the border with Chile. (Google, n. d.).

prescriptions, vaccinate, perform pregnancy and healthy children surveillance, and also provide primary care before ambulance arrival in case of emergencies). Considering the long distances and geographic characteristics of this region,

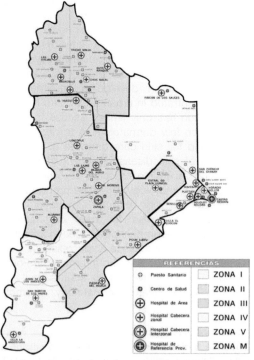

Fig. 2. Neuquén Province sanitary division with different levels of complexity. (Neuquen Province Government, Sept 2014).

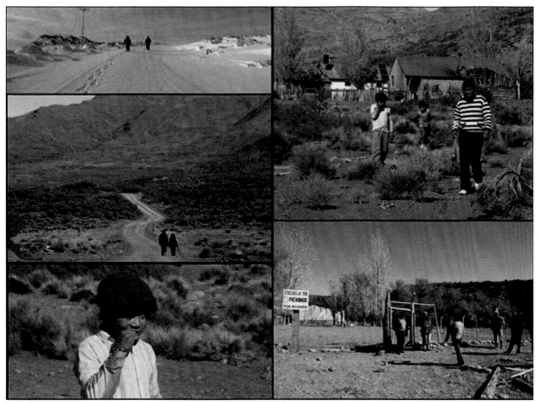

Fig. 3. In rural areas, patients need to walk long distances in different climate conditions to attend the monthly hospital visit.

primary care agents play a key role in the first level of medical attention (**Fig. 4**).

RECIPIENTS

Educating general physicians in prevalent skin diseases was one of our primary goals, and at the beginning we designed all our activities focusing on them as the main recipients. However, over time we realized that medical students and other health personnel, and particularly the community in general, have been willing to receive educational activities. Including medical students in this kind of program provides important dermatologic education, which is not usually covered in the regular medical school curricula and makes it possible for them to participate in a humanitarian interdisciplinary experience, which may be a nice model to replicate in their future careers independently of the specialization they choose.

DESIGN CHARACTERISTICS OF THE PROGRAM

When designing any health community program, some important qualities should be taken into account. These are discussed next.

Adequacy

Community dermatology programs should be adequate for the community and health workers of the area. Previous knowledge of the people and community is required, according to intercultural concepts. One example is that Mapuche communities, as many other subsistence producers, have a special relationship with the sun, because it is closely related to the prosperity of their plantations and animals. Ignoring this when designing a photoeducational workshop may hurt their feelings, and thus we cannot start the activity by simply saying that "the sun is bad for our health."

Stability/Replicability

Performing activities that can be replicated with the same structure in different locations makes it possible to collect epidemiologic data, assess impact, and share ideas for improvement from different communities. Our activities are being replicated in Uruguay, Chile, and the north of Argentina (Jujuy). Not every model works in every environment, so each group should adapt the

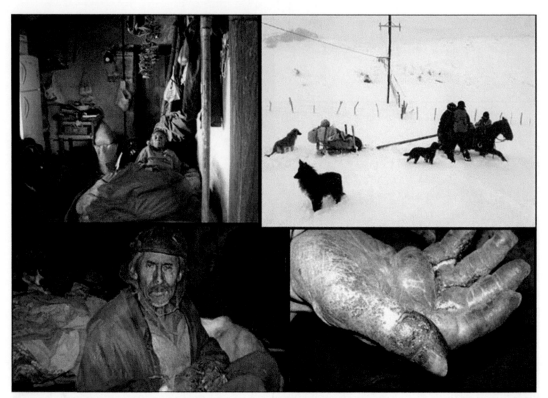

Fig. 4. Sometimes leaving the rural area is not so easy. (*Top*) Mario Merino (nurse) helps with sleigh transportation of a lady with pneumonia. (*Bottom*) An old man with burn injuries in his hands could not leave his house for 1 week before receiving any medical attention.

activities to the most practical and effective way for each environment.

Simplicity

Activities should aim to require minimal human/economic resources, because available funding is typically limited. In our program, some activities are simple and can be performed by one person (photoeducational workshops, atopic dermatitis workshops). Other activities, such as the *jornadas*, are more complex and varied, depending on the financial and human resources available.

Continuity/Sustainability

The persistence of the project throughout time should run independently of specific health personnel.

Flexibility

The program should be adaptable to changing variables, such as adverse weather, sociopolitical crises, participants numbers, and community size.

Positivity

As a priority, the activities should aim to be imbued with a joyful spirit. If people taking part in these activities, who rely on their free time to do so, do not experience a positive attitude, a heavy drain on human resources will, sooner or later, become apparent. We firmly believe that the enthusiasm and passion displayed by the group is the most "essential" fuel that keeps any community dermatology project alive.

ENDORSEMENTS AND STAKEHOLDERS

- *International Foundation for Dermatology*. The collaboration of the International Foundation for Dermatology was crucial for the program's development, through three development grants (2013–2019), which allowed Dr Casas to receive in-person training and continued support.
- *Neuquén Province Public Health System*. All the activities are organized and promoted within the Ministry of Health of the Neuquén province, which does not provide funding, but is important to facilitate interinstitutional cooperation.
- *Comahue National University Faculty of Medicine*. Since 2014, the project is included as one of the Extension University Programs of Comahue National University. The program

enlists volunteers from the fifth year of medical school to fulfill a 3-month course in ultraviolet radiation (UVR) carcinogenesis. At the end of the course, the students perform photoeducational workshops in primary schools in the university area.

- *American Academy of Dermatology*. In August 2014, Dr Casas received the American Academy of Dermatology "Members Making a Difference" award in recognition of her outstanding volunteer service and dedication in this labor.
- Both the *Argentinian Association of Dermatology* and the *Argentinian Society of Dermatology* gave institutional endorsement to the project, not including economic support.

ACTIVITIES INCLUDED IN THE PROGRAM
Jornadas

The *jornadas* are massive free-of-charge dermatology clinics for communities, where volunteer dermatologists see a large number of patients while teaching local practitioners at the same time (**Fig. 5**). The *jornadas* are a highly visible activity with an important added political value: they solve skin problems of people in the community. This health care activity allows people from cities with no access to a dermatologist to be assessed by a group of specialists together with their local doctors. Physicians and health care workers receive education in prevalent skin diseases and learn how to care for their own patients, whereas people from distant communities receive free dermatologic consultation. The main goal of the program is educational: we strongly consider education is the most effective way of producing long-term changes in skin health in these remote areas (**Fig. 6**).

The main objective is training local health care workers in the diagnosis and management of prevalent dermatologic pathologies. Following the dermatology clinic, lectures are given in a workshop format, focusing on diagnostic tools, how to triage severity/need for referral, therapeutic options, and skin biopsy technique. In one session, local practitioners can present their own challenging cases. In another, patients seen at the *jornada* are discussed as a group (**Fig. 7**). These activities are highly valuable, because volunteer dermatologists actively share their own expertise among each other for group learning. The epidemiologic data obtained are shared with all the participants, allowing different lines of investigation.

The *jornadas* have been held in rural areas of Neuquén province twice per year since 2009, and they have been replicated in other provinces by local dermatologists that learned from volunteering in Patagonia (**Table 1**).

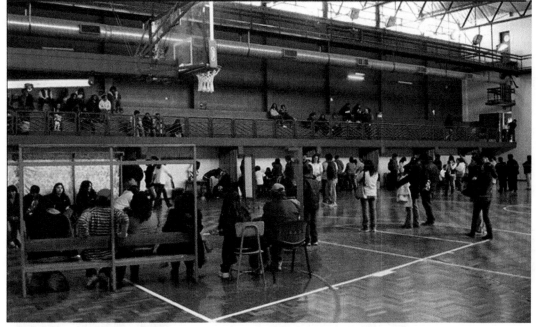

Fig. 5. At each *jornada* in Argentina, several offices are set up in gyms or school buildings, providing dermatologic consultation to an average of 120 patients. Chos Malal, 2013.

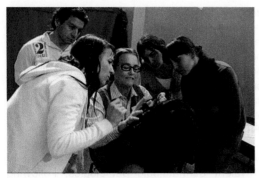

Fig. 6. Dr Juliana Förster Fernandez gives consultation accompanied by local physicians and health care workers. Chos Malal, 2013.

Legal framework

In Argentina, medical practice is under provincial regulation, and a registration is required to practice. There are antecedents of itinerant medicine in government and nongovernmental organizations, which are often run without regulation. In contrast, our program is endorsed by the Ministry of Health of the province and the local hospitals where each *jornadas* take place. The professionals invited to participate are accompanied by local doctors authorized for medical practice in the province. We use an exception that endorses medical practice in the public sector for a limited time under the supervision of competent professionals (Art. 17132).[12]

Ethical considerations

Using local health service providers allows continuity to the health care process, long-term accountability and availability, the best interpretation of local peculiarities, and achievement of higher therapeutic adherence. Itinerant professionals should not be seen as competitors but as part of the team, reinforcing the existing health care capacity and creating networks to access needed specialty consultation (in person or virtual). This encourages health care continuity, professional collaboration, teamwork, and therapeutic compliance.

To uphold patient rights, the features and limitations of the facility are explained before the patient encounter. Because these are massive events, the facilities lack typical medical equipment. We ensure everyone involved is a health care personnel (under confidentiality agreement) and that private areas are secured for patient care when needed. Care is always provided together with local representatives for a streamlined process allowing specialists to understand local resources to maximize results and reinforce therapeutic compliance.[13]

Teledermatology

There is an official teledermatology platform endorsed by the Public Health Ministry of Neuquén province created in 2013 with the expertise advice of Dr Karen McKoy (USA). Regular consultations are also made in daily practice using more familiar mobile phone applications, such as WhatsApp. Medical officers and health care workers attending the *jornadas* are encouraged to maintain e-mail or WhatsApp connection with the dermatologists participating in the project, to receive supervision

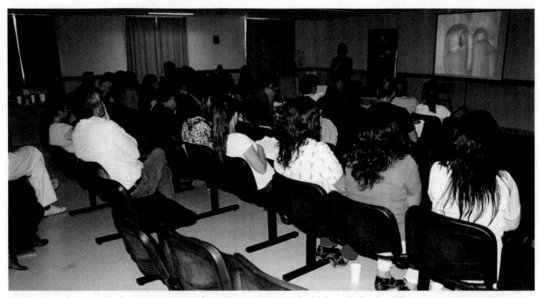

Fig. 7. At each *jornada*, lectures on prevalent dermatosis are held for all the health personnel attending.

Table 1
Jornadas performed between 2009 and 2019, summarizing volunteering dermatologists and recipients of each activity

	Dermatologists Volunteering	Health Care Workers Attending	Children Attending Workshops	Patients Seen
Chos Malal 2010	7	51	497	262
JDA 2010	8	72	37	64
VLA 2011	10	60	27	80
Chos Malal 2011	14	54	500	392
LC/Aluminé 2011	17	46	144	471
SMA2012	5	89	135	72
Zapala 2012	11	50	78	261
Centenario 2013	7	72	43	96
Chos Malal 2013	8	45	—	272
Loncopue 2014	3	6	19	18
Centenario 2015	5	42	26	63
SMA/LC 2016	4	8	26	36
JDA 2016	3	6	—	15
Bahía Blanca 2017	12	53	27	112
SMA workshops 2017	1	16	726	24
Montevideo 2017	3	—	64	—
Jujuy 2017	4	42	127	63
Las Lajas 2018	5	22	120	96
Jujuy 2018	3	16	120	45
Atacama 2018	2	8	70	—
SMA 2018	7	47	26	120
Montevideo 2017	10		16 schools	
Total		805	2812	2562

on patient follow-up. The first face-to-face encounter at a *jornada* allows a more familiar and colloquial relationship through the teledermatology platform in the future. An average of 30 teledermatology consultations is performed monthly.

Photoeducational Workshops

Mapuche communities in the Cordillera de los Andes live in high mountain landscapes where sun exposure is strong during many hours and humidity is extremely low, with windy weather and extreme temperatures.[14] According to the epidemiologic data surveyed during the *jornadas* between 2009 and 2019, sun and dry skin related dermatoses (rosacea, actinic prurigo, melasma, atopic dermatitis, and others) accounted for 70% of skin pathologies detected in mountain areas (**Fig. 8**). We selected on sun-related skin conditions for educational activities because, with proper education, general physicians can manage

them to generate significant improvements in patient outcomes.

We focused on two community groups that would benefit from this education: children younger than 8 and advanced medical students. Through feedback from teachers, these workshops have evolved throughout the years. At the beginning they were performed by one person, in the classic expository lecture format. An extraordinary teacher, Patricia Renee Frete, who is also theater director and hospital clown, joined our permanent team, and provided us with her invaluable educational expertise and assistance. The activity has since adopted the characteristics of a brief theater play with one character as the "doctor" and the second character as "the assistant," who performs funny interactions with children, making every workshop a unique product.

The structure of the workshop is clearly divided into three parts. The first part is a typical lecture from a professor; however, we engage students

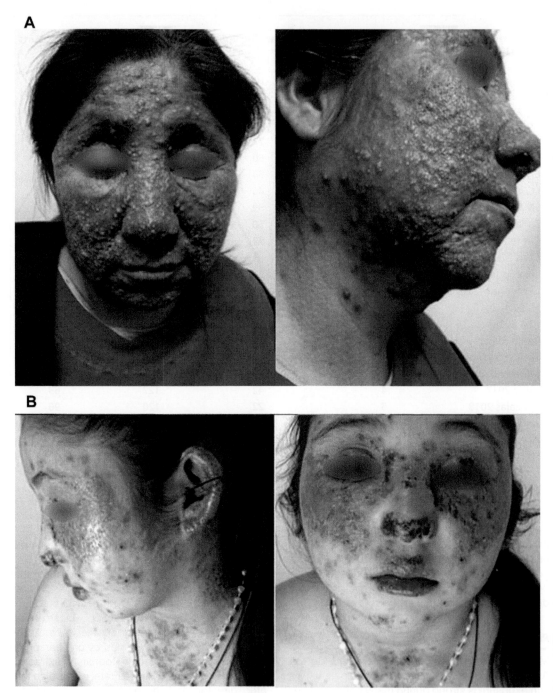

Fig. 8. Two cases of severe actinic prurigo. (*A*) Aggravated by the overuse of corticoid creams. (*B*) Acute vesico-bullous form, more frequent in children.

by giving them idea that the assistant, Azucena, is in charge and supposed to give the lecture. The professor character appears worried and tells the children that he will have to present the workshop instead because his/her assistant is late. The lecture must be less than 15 minutes to avoid boredom or distraction. The contents should be simple and concise, focusing on basic concepts: (1) the sun is a star that produces energy that makes life possible but can also be harmful in excess, producing sunburns, aging, and skin diseases; (2) our planet has an effective shield, the atmosphere, but it does not work so efficiently at midday, so if we take care of the time of the day for outdoor activities, we would receive little of the "bad" sun; and (3) there are other things that protect us, such as wide-brim hats, long sleeve clothes, sunglasses, and sunscreens that also contribute greatly by reducing the amount of UVR that reaches our skin (**Fig. 9**).

The second part begins just at the time children are reaching their attention limit: the abrupt entrance of the second character, Azucena, who is arriving late to the activity and makes the professor angry. A small discussion among the two characters takes place, and surprise renews the childrens' attention. Azucena begs the professor to let her present the workshop she has missed for being late. A telephone call interrupts this dialogue and the professor is forced to leave the room. The professor leaves, saying that he/she will be back in a moment and will ask Azucena some questions about the contents presented. Azucena is then left alone with the kids, and almost in tears starts begging the children to help her by telling her all the information the professor had just told them. This is the most effective pedagogic tool of the workshop: children use the information to help another person. Putting them in a position to reiterate the contents recently delivered to them to another person (Azucena) is a brain plasticity process that promotes lasting learning (**Fig. 10**).

The third part of the workshop starts when the professor returns and asks questions to Azucena as an oral examination. Azucena answers questions in a funny way, using impressive visual tools (eg, a huge inflatable sun with two faces [a smiling one and angry looking one] to show the different intensities of UVR at different times of the day, black elastic socks to represent the different length of shadows, a small useless hat compared with a super-giant Mexican hat) (**Fig. 11**).

The repetition of the contents including games and visual accessories at the end is another highly

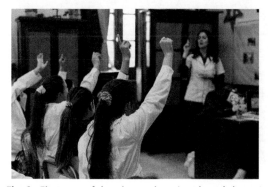

Fig. 9. First part of the photoeducational workshop. A regular lecture providing basic concepts about different UVR indexes at different times of the day.

effective pedagogic tool making the activity emotional and memorable for the children. Each child receives a simple positive memory of the activity to take home and recall in the future (**Fig. 12**). Parents, teachers, nurses, and generalist doctors usually watch the workshop: the simplicity, pedagogic and didactic way of explaining the sun's effects on our skin, and the different protection alternatives also reach the adults with a stronger impact than a complicated and complex dissertation on UVR.

Photoeducational workshops have demonstrated to be a simple, easy to perform, funny for children and adults, successful, and memorable activity that leaves everyone with a joyful feeling. Making kids laugh has shown to be a fast and effective way of obtaining local community approval and health care workers' confidence, which is one of the most difficult challenges of community dermatology programs: reaching a community as a whole.

Videos of photoeducational workshop fragments available at: https://www.youtube.com/watch?v=vu9Paut3C24 and https://www.youtube.com/watch?v=ZqJRzs98quU&t=1s.

Community workshops pedagogic tips
Neuroscience and developmental cognitive research focuses on understanding the neurobiologic basis of learning.[15] Little is known about how such processes as learning and memory evolve from early childhood throughout adolescence. It is known that learning is influenced by the emotional context, the environment, and individual differences.[16] It is also known that interaction with the world takes place through the senses, and each sense uses parallel ways: what is read, what is heard, what is touched, and so forth. The final result of things we perceive is the "construction" made by our brain with all that information obtained through different sensorial ways, in addition to added emotional content. All these facts increasingly oppose traditional pedagogy, which centers on the professor as the main actor of the educational process.

Awareness of the different types of memory storage can optimize teaching techniques. What makes certain content stored as short- versus long-term memory is still under investigation. However, it is known, among other variables, that the use of information as a tool to perform a productive, playful, or pleasant activity soon after its reception is related to a higher capacity to hold that information as long-term memory. In our workshops for children, making them active participants in the learning process allows them to give meaning to the information received, thus

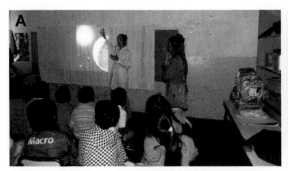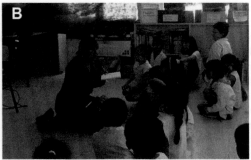

Fig. 10. Second part of the photoeducational workshop. After the surprise of her entrance (*A*), the assistant, Azucena, is left alone with the kids and asks for their help in refreshing all the concepts they have just received (*B*).

increasing the chance for that information to be stored long-term.[17] This empathic, face-to-face meeting, between student and teacher is a key pedagogic mediation in educational action.[18] Designing this type of activity is difficult, although highly stimulating because it recovers interest in teaching and interest in learning.[19] It creates communication bridges that provide parents, educators, and health care personnel a simple, memorable, fun, and highly effective way of teaching.

Photoeducational workshops expansion
We have sought to develop new approaches to maximize the audience reached in more school environments.

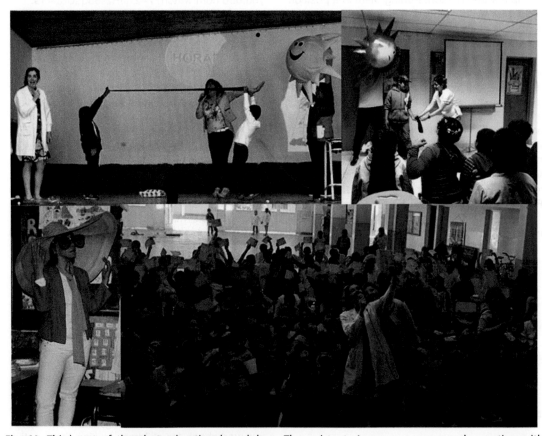

Fig. 11. Third part of the photoeducational workshop. The assistant, Azucena, answers each question with impressive visual accessories. In the end all the group takes a selfie with a vintage line telephone creating a magic moment of imaginative play with the kids.

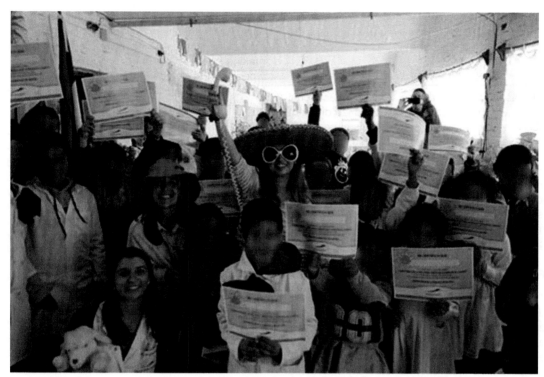

Fig. 12. Children receive colorful Skin Scientist Diplomas with their names on them. Uruguay 2018.

In 2014 the Faculty of Medicine of the Comahue National Medical University approved an Extension Program for fifth-year medical students to form part of the photoeducational workshops project, consisting of three steps: (1) lectures on skin anatomy and physiology, skin cancer, UVR, photoprotection, and sunscreens; (2) brief training on theatrical techniques and pedagogic tips for children's activities; and (3) in groups of five to six, students performing their own photoeducatlonal workshops in at least three different schools. The aim of the Extension University program is that medical students gain interest in developing primary care activities in dermatology and educating children in their own community. Students had provided feedback on hoping for the opportunity to learn more about skin cancer than their brief 2-week dermatology curriculum in medical school. They also highlighted that helping the community by doing some medical work while they were still student doctors gave them a good feeling. Student training in developing community workshops is an important tool that may be used later for other health issues. This innovative extracurricular activity provides special skills that may be useful in their future medical work.

Since 2016 Dr Luz Daje is replicating photoeducational workshops with local teachers in cooperation with the Ministry of Education of Jujuy (North of Argentina).

Since 2018 Dr Maria Eugenia Mazzei has developed photoeducational workshops with the Uruguay Clinicas Hospital and these have become a regular activity of the Dermatology Residency Program of Uruguay. Second-year dermatology residents receive 2-week training in photoeducational workshops at San Martin de los Andes, and then they replicate the work in rural Uruguay. Nine departments have been visited to impact 628 children.[20]

Atopic Dermatitis Workshops

Inspired by photoeducational workshops, Dr Maria Eugenia Mazzei from Uruguay created a version aimed at atopic dermatitis. It shares the same three-part structure but it is adapted to this unique condition. The atopic dermatitis workshop focuses on skin care by giving simple and daily tips to improve health. Patients with atopic dermatitis feel much better after the workshops, because they can interact with others sharing the condition who experience similar concerns and problems. Pediatricians attending the workshops get familiarized with gentle skin care techniques that are often more important than prescription medications but are not always emphasized in scientific literature. Because the workshop is aimed at children, simple language is well received to make the activity funny and memorable.

Photoeducational World Wide Web Video

To reach a larger audience, a short educational video was produced and uploaded at different public health Web sites. The video is aimed at 8- to 10-year-old children and intended to be used by any health care worker interested in photoeducational projects. It should be shown after a brief introductory talk about the solar system, and followed by some exercises and games. The video is free for any nonprofit educational activity, mentioning the source, at https://www.youtube.com/watch?v=mzaHSa8ghKw.

FUTURE OF THE PROGRAM

The project will continue performing *jornadas* in different places of Argentina depending on the economic resources available. Photoeducational and atopic dermatitis workshop scripts are available to be shared with any scientific society or health-related Web site, so that any interested dermatologist or health care worker is able to use them. We want to develop more workshops for other prevalent dermatosis in our region, such as pediculosis, scabies, and rosacea; and share the model to be used for any other prevalent dermatosis in other parts of the world.

DISCUSSION

We believe in education as the most effective and long-lasting strategy to obtain sustainable improvements in community health. We, dermatologists, talk in many scientific meetings, but we seldom organize activities aimed at medical students or the wider community. The disproportion between the number of events for dermatologists and events aimed at the community is expansive. After significant discussion, we seem to have forgotten to teach basic dermatology directly to the community. Mastering a certain topic does not ensure the capability to teach. Medical discourse is anchored in a hermetic language, sometimes incomprehensible even for specialists themselves, as is the case with the "argument from authority" (which is based on using such a technical discourse that just a hundred specialists can understand and judge what is being presented).[21] It is not about making a bad quality diffusion with poor scientific value, but rather having the best experts on certain topics produce excellent scientific-level material, developed with a simple, accessible-to-all, "free of formalisms" language, using basic and every day analogies without distorting the content. Simplifying content without making them banal not only prevents overwhelming the audience but also encourages attendants to acquire further knowledge in this new field of study presented in a friendly way.

Decisions on what to teach, when, how, and to whom should be made after a thorough preanalysis to avoid wasting resources and time. Pedagogues, school boards, ministries of health and education, local health workers, and the scientific community should work in an interdisciplinary way to plan educational strategies appropriately and thus obtain the best results. In our case, educational activities were originally meant for general physicians, but as time went by, medical students, nurses, health care workers, and especially small children and the community became the most important recipients of the program.

Organizing massive free-of-charge dermatology clinics in the context of a 2-day intensive training period is a highly visible and politically profitable activity; but it requires major funding, many people involved, and a strong support and endorsement from different institutions (eg, public health system, university, scientific societies). We strongly recommend that patients should always be seen together with local health workers; otherwise, the activity is only a welfarism action with no pedagogic legacy.

At present, working directly with the community through workshops for children at primary schools, performed by dermatology residents, medical students, and general medicine residents is our most cost-effective enjoyable activity, which can be performed involving one or two people, with few resources, and with no need of a big institutional structure.

The *jornadas* and the community workshops (photoeducational and atopic dermatitis workshops) are our two main strategies to bridge the gap between distant poor communities and trained dermatologists. The benefits of these strategies are hard to estimate, and short-, medium-, and long-term impact evaluation programs need to be designed and established.

REFERENCES

1. Hay RJ, Estrada R, Grossmann H. Managing skin disease in recourse-poor environments: the role of community-oriented training and control programs. Int J Dermatol 2011;50:558–63.
2. Hay RJ, Andersson N, Estrada R. Mexico: community dermatology in Guerrero. Lancet 1991;337:906–7.

3. Available at: https://ilds.org/our-foundation/. Accessed September 6, 2020.

4. Available at: https://gloderm.org. Accessed September 6, 2020.

5. Kopf AW. International Foundation for Dermatology. A challenge to meet the dermatologic needs of developing countries. Dermatol Clin 1993;II:311–4.

6. Available at: http://rdtc.go.tz/about-us/history/. Accessed September 6, 2020.

7. Available at: http://www.dermatologiacomunitaria.org.mx/somos.html. Accessed September 6, 2020.

8. National Census 2010, Dirección Provincial de Estadísticas y Censos, Provincia del Neuquen. Available at: https://estadisticaneuquen.gob.ar. Accessed August 1, 2019.

9. Hay RJ. Dermatologic primary care program for Neuquen Province, Patagonia, Argentina. J Comm Dermatol 2011;7:1–2.

10. Hay R. Dermatologic Primary Care Programme for Neuquén Province, Patagonia, Argentina. J Comm Dermatol 2011;7:1–2. Available at: https://ilds.org/wp-content/uploads/2018/04/Community_Dermatology_11_.pdf. Accessed September 6, 2020.

11. Hay RJ, Buxton P. The International Foundation for Dermatology and community dermatology. J Comm Dermatol 2009;6:13–5.

12. Riccardini JC. Ejercicio Ilegal de la Medicina. Buenos Aires, Argentina: Asociación del Pensamiento Penal; 2013. Available at: http://www.pensamientopenal.com.ar/system/files/cpcomentado/cpc37772.pdf. Accessed August 1, 2019.

13. Aguirre-Gas H. La ética y la calidad de atención médica. Cir medical 2002;70:50–4. Available at: https://www.medigraphic.com/cgi-bin/new/resumen.cgi?IDARTICULO=3184.

14. Casas IMP. Sun protection and actinic dermatosis in rural communities. World Dermatology Meeting 2019, Milan. Humanitarian Dermatology Session. Abstract. Available at: https://www.wcd2019milan-dl.org/abstract-book/documents/invited-speakers-abstracts/20-humanitarian-dermatology-migrant-health/sun-protection-and-actinic-dermatitis-76.pdf. Accessed September 6, 2020.

15. Ferreira TJM. Neurociencia + Pedagogía = Neuropedagogía: Repercusiones e Implicaciones de los Avances de la Neurociencia para la Práctica Educativa. Tesina: Universidad Internacional de Andalucía; 2012. Available at: https://dspace.unia.es/bitstream/handle/10334/2075/0341_Ferreira.pdf?sequence=1. Accessed August 1, 2019.

16. Freire P. Educación como práctica de la libertad. 2a edición. Buenos Aires (Argentina): Siglo XXI Editores Argentina; 2008.

17. Blakemore SJ, Frith U. The learning brain. Oxford (England): Blackwell Publishing Ltd; 2007.

18. Prieto Castillo D, Gutiérrez Pérez F. La mediación Pedagógica. Buenos Aires (Argentina): La Crujía; 2007.

19. Litwin E. El oficio de enseñar: Condiciones y Contextos. Buenos Aires (Argentina): Paidós; 2009.

20. Mazzei ME, Casas IMP. Community dermatology: a bi-national project. Poster at WDC, Milan 2019. Available at: https://www.wcd2019milan-dl.org/abstract-book/documents/abstracts/16-global-skin-health/community-dermatology-a-bi-national-1988.pdf. Accessed September 6, 2020.

21. Schiff M. A inteligência desperdiçada: desigualdade social, injustiça escolar. Porto Alegre. Artes Médicas 1994;43–4.

Dermatology Training in Africa: Successes and Challenges

Anisa Mosam, MB ChB, FC Derm (SA), MMed (Derm), PhD (UKZN)[a,b,*],
Gail Todd, BSc (Agric), MB ChB, FF Derm (SA), PhD (UCT)[c]

KEYWORDS

- Dermatology training • Dermatology education • Dermato-venereology training
- Dermato-venereology education • Curricula • Africa

KEY POINTS

- In North Africa, the ratio of dermatologists ranges from 3 per million population to 49 per million population. The rest of the continent has a ratio less than 10 per million population, usually less than 1 per million population. Inadequate numbers of dermatologists to disease burden needs task shifting to provide service.
- Of the 55 African countries, 30 countries have no training programs, 12 have a regional program, 8 have a national program, and 5 have university programs.
- Training programs emphasize modern biomedical treatments and the latest therapies, which have limited availability, are neither cost-effective nor based on evidence from Africa or skin of color.
- Current health systems in Africa respond to causes of death but not the long-term effects of health conditions and associated functional limitations.
- Pooling of expertise and resources is necessary to strengthen training and develop curricula relevant to local African needs.

INTRODUCTION

Africa has a population of 1.2 billion, with a population density of 30.5 people per square kilometer.[1] Its 55 countries are grouped into 5 regions by the African Union.[2] A literature review of English language epidemiology publications from 1970 to 2005 by the World Health Organization reported that the prevalence of skin disease and their associated morbidity in African countries (6 studies) ranges from 26.9% (Tanzania, 2 rural villages) to 80.4% (Ethiopia, 1 rural village).[3] Incidence data of skin disease in the general population were scarce. Four studies reported on the frequency of new consultations for skin disease in primary health in Africa, which ranged from 6.9% (Mali, all levels of public health care) to 13% (Cameroon, 83 villages primary care).[3]

Earlier attempts to describe strategies for dermatology training in Africa focused predominantly on anglophone countries and noted that specialist training was limited.[4]

The ratio of dermatologists to populations in Africa is speculative and needs formal evaluation. Most African dermatologists practice as private practitioners in urban areas. Only a minority are in academic and public service. This results in limited to absent skin health care for large sectors of the population.[5]

A survey of dermato-venereology education and service provision on the continent is thus timely.

POSTGRADUATE DERMATOLOGY TRAINING PROGRAMS IN AFRICA

This section is based on information received from dermatologists in academic positions

[a] Department of Dermatology, University of KwaZulu-Natal, Durban, South Africa Rm 327, 3rd Floor, Main Building, Durban, South Africa; [b] Nelson R Mandela School of Medicine, 719 Umbilo Rd, 4013, Durban, South Africa; [c] Department of Medicine, Faculty of Health Sciences, University of Cape Town, Anzio Road, Observatory 7925, Cape Town, South Africa
* Corresponding author.
E-mail address: Mosama@ukzn.ac.za

Dermatol Clin 39 (2021) 57–71
https://doi.org/10.1016/j.det.2020.08.006
0733-8635/21/© 2020 Elsevier Inc. All rights reserved.

across the continent supplemented with information obtained from the internet, publications, and personal experience. Academics at institutions in most countries across Africa were approached as well as the Association of African Universities. Most requests for information on training programs and curricula were received positively and information provided; however, there are information gaps in some regions. Rudimentary data from some programs have been included where possible, even though complete discussion of the respective programs was not possible. There may also be programs that inadvertently have been overlooked.

TRAINING PROGRAMS IN VARIOUS REGIONS IN AFRICA
Southern Africa

The countries of Southern Africa are Angola, Botswana, Eswatini, Lesotho, Malawi, Mozambique, Namibia, South Africa, Zambia, and Zimbabwe.

South Africa and Mozambique were the only countries in this region where training programs could be identified.

South Africa
South Africa is the fifth most populous country in Africa. It has a population of 59.3 million, with 177 dermatologists.

There are 8 universities, each with a health care faculty and dermatology training program. The universities and associated teaching hospitals are responsible for the teaching of dermatology residents. The national curriculum and examinations for specialist training are provided by the College of Dermatologists of the Colleges of Medicine of South Africa (CMSA). Forty resident training posts paid for by the Department of Health are distributed across the 8 universities. Supernumerary residents who are self-funded are also trained.

Registration as a medical doctor by the accrediting body, the Health Professions Council of South Africa is the sole entry requirement. There is no national/central system of appointments. The posts are competitive, and each university has its own preferences. Residents entering the system have 4 years in which to complete their specialist training. Two national examinations are held twice a year under the auspices of the CMSA. Part 1, taken after 1 year of residency, examines the basic sciences relevant to dermatology, and Part 2 is the exit clinical examination. A portfolio of learning and in-course continuous assessment are compulsory requirements for the Fellowship of the College of Dermatologists (FC Derm [SA]) of the CMSA. A

minithesis must be completed in the 4 years of training and is an essential additional requirement for the MMed degree.

For registration as an independent dermatologist, the national FC Derm (SA) exit examination, training time of a minimum of 4 years in an accredited training facility, and MMed in dermatology are required.

Additional training is available in dermatologic surgery and Mohs surgery, through the South African Society of Dermatological Surgery and a Mohs fellowship that is accredited by the American Academy of Dermatology (**Box 1**).

North Africa

The countries of North Africa are Algeria, Egypt, Libya, Mauritania, Morocco, Tunisia, and Western Sahara (Sahrawi Arab Democratic Republic).

Aside from Algeria, Egypt, Libya, Morocco, and Tunisia, the authors have been unable to establish details of training programs in the other countries (**Box 2**).

Egypt
Egypt has a population of 102.3 million, serviced by 5000 dermatologists, the highest number on the continent.

There are 20 national universities and 4 private universities offering postgraduate teaching programs. There is a Ministry of Health Egyptian Fellowship, which is a national program of 5 years, and each university has its own master's (MSc) 3-year program and examination, which follow the national curriculum but with some flexibility. A clinical PhD of 5 years' duration is also offered and the 3-year masters can be upgraded to a 5-year fellowship or clinical PhD. The curricula and exit examinations differ between universities, but in all masters programs a logbook must be

---

Box 1
Key facts for Southern Africa

- Dermatologist/million country inhabitants varies from 0 to 3 (**Figs. 1** and **2**) and all practice in urban areas.

- The 4-year specialist fellowship in South Africa, FC Derm (SA), has a national curriculum and examination by College of Dermatologists of South Africa. For the university-based MMed, a thesis is required. To register as a specialist dermatologist, both the FC Derm (SA) and MMed are required

- The Mozambique qualification is a 5-year diploma in dermato-venereology with 3 years of the 5 years spent in dermatology.

Box 2
Key facts for North Africa

- Dermatologist/million country inhabitants varies from 3 in Mauritania to 49 in Egypt (see **Figs. 1** and **2**).
- The highest number of practicing dermatologists (5000) is found in Egypt.
- Egypt offers a 5-year master's program with MD/PhD.
- Libya and Tunisia have a 4-year master's program with exit examination.
- Details from the Algerian and Moroccan programs were unavailable at the time of publication.

completed by the students. A thesis is required for the PhD (MD) program, not the master's (MSc).

Approximately 4 resident positions become available yearly in each university, so approximately 100 residents per year are chosen based on the Bachelor of Medicine and Bachelor of Surgery (MBChB) degree and academic grades. University diplomas in focused specialization areas are offered for laser and aesthetic dermatology and require additional training periods.

Libya

Libya has a population of 6.9 million, with 80 dermatologists. The educational and training program in dermatology in Libya comprises 2 different specialty programs, both of which have a selection examination.

The master's degree (MSc) in dermatology and venereology is a university degree awarded by the Faculty of Medicine, Benghazi University. It is a 2-year program with theory and a practical that involves a Part I examination on basic sciences and a Part II on clinical dermatology. There is also a thesis component.

The Libyan board degree in dermatology and venereology (medical doctorate) is awarded by the Libyan Board of Medical Specialties. It is a 4-year training program with theory and practical components, where training is documented in a logbook. In addition to dermatology, the training includes 9 months of rotations in rheumatology, endocrinology, infectious diseases, plastic surgery, hematology pediatrics, and pathology.

The examination includes 2 parts. Part I is a written examination after 1 year of training, mainly in basic dermatology and allied disciplines like plastic surgery and rheumatology. The thesis can be started after passing Part I. The Part II examination is written at the end of training and involves a written and a practical examined by internal and external examiners.

Tunisia

For a population of 11.8 million in Tunisia, there are 420 dermatologists. Currently there are 4 medical schools in Tunisia (Tunis, Sousse, Sfax, and Monastir) and 7 departments of dermatology, 1 being the Armed Forces Hospital. Military dermatologists are fully integrated in the teaching of dermatology in Tunis Medical School. There is a national curriculum accredited by the College of Dermatology, La Société Tunisienne de Dermatologie et de Vénéréologie.[6]

To join dermatology, candidates must pass a national residency examination, and those who are ranked highest are offered posts. There were 12 open positions for dermatology residency in 2019; the last one who was offered a training position ranked 30 out of 1000. The 4-year training program is divided into 8 separate 6-month rotations as follows: 6 compulsory semesters of dermatology and 2 optional semesters in either internal medicine, pathologic anatomy, pediatrics, maxillofacial surgery, genetics, pharmacology, immunology, and dermatology or parasitology. During training, Tunisian residents may rotate in dermatology departments outside Tunisia for more exposure to skin diseases. No thesis or portfolio is required but publications are encouraged, especially if residents want to enter the academic sphere. The national examination takes place once a year and is arranged by the Ministry of Health and Higher Education; examiners are chosen by the Ministry of Health. The examination involves a theory paper, clinical cases, and a discussion of research outputs. To become a specialist, a national examination must be passed, taken after 4 years of residency.

Approximately 16 new Tunisian dermatologists graduate yearly in Tunisia. A similar number of Tunisians graduate from programs in Romania, Ukraine, Russia, and Senegal. On returning to Tunisia, these foreign-trained Tunisian dermatologists must spend additional time in local training and pass an examination for their qualification to be recognized as equivalent to the Tunisian training.

West Africa

The countries of West Africa are Benin, Burkina Faso, Cabo Verde, Côte d'Ivoire, The Gambia, Ghana, Guinea-Conakry, Guinea-Bissau, Liberia, Mali, Niger, Nigeria, Senegal, Sierra Leone, and Togo.

The authors have been able to establish details of training programs only in Nigeria, Mali, Senegal, and Ghana (**Box 3**).

Ghana

Ghana, a rapidly developing West African country of 31.1 million people, is served by 33 certified dermatologists. In conjunction with the Ghana College of Physicians and Surgeons, the Ghana Society of Dermatology established Ghana's first and only dermatology training fellowship at Korle-Bu Teaching Hospital, the largest public hospital in Accra, in 2012.

They follow the harmonized curriculum for the West African region. This 5-year supervised training program requires a logbook to document training experiences and a research component in the form of a thesis. There is also an exit examination. Currently there is no subspecialty training.

Mali

Mali is the eighth largest country in Africa, with a population of 20.3 million. Mali currently has 30 certified dermatologists and 16 residents in training. The Mali dermatology training program is based on the harmonized curriculum for West African countries.

Nigeria

Nigeria is the most populous country in Africa, with a population of 206.1 million and the fastest growth rate.[1] There are 132 dermatologists in Nigeria, concentrated mostly in the largest cities.

Dermato-venereology is considered a subspecialty of internal medicine. Dermatology training follows the harmonized curriculum of the Postgraduate Medical Colleges in the West African subregion. There are 2 national colleges for residency training, the National Postgraduate Medical College of Nigeria and the West African College of Physicians. Dermato-venereology candidates are admitted for the 5-year fellowship after completion of the undergraduate qualification and 2 years in internal medicine or its subspecialties. Part 1 of the fellowship involves an examination in internal medicine. Approximately 45 residents go on to complete a further 3 years of dedicated dermatology rotations to finish their dermatology training. They then sit for a national fellowship examination in dermatology held twice a year. A logbook documenting their supervised progress and a dissertation also are required.

Senegal

Senegal has a population of 16.7 million and 54 dermatologists. A national program for specialization in dermatology started in the late 1990s and is of 4 years' duration. The fourth year is dedicated to research with a thesis and oral defense, required to obtain the diploma of Specialist in Dermatology.

East Africa

The countries of East Africa are Comoros, Djibouti, Eritrea, Ethiopia, Kenya, Madagascar, Mauritius, Rwanda, Seychelles, Somalia, South Sudan, Sudan, Tanzania, and Uganda.

The authors have been able to establish details of training programs only in Tanzania, Ethiopia, Kenya, Madagascar, and Uganda (**Box 4**).

Ethiopia

Ethiopia is the second most populous country in Africa, with a population of 115 million people. There are 100 dermato-venereologists in the country.

Dermatology training programs were initiated in 2006 and initially based at Addis Ababa and Mekelle Universities. Due to gaps in these curricula, a national harmonized curriculum was developed by the Technical Working Group for dermato-venereology under the direction of the Ministry of Health, Human Resource Development Directorate. The Technical Working Group members are experienced trainers from Ethiopia, with special expertise in different areas of dermato-venereology. Feedback has been obtained from members of the Ethiopian Dermatology and Venereology Society and others with expertise in teaching dermatology. This curriculum defines specialty training leading to a certificate of completion of training in dermatology and venereology and is now established in 6 institutions nationally. The curriculum covers the acquisition of all competencies required for a consultant dermato-venereologist practicing in Ethiopia. To be enrolled in the program, candidates must take the national resident matching examination for selection to the approximately 26 training positions annually. Residents are also accepted from neighboring countries, such as Somalia and South Sudan.

The 3-year training program follows a spiral curriculum covering basic sciences and all aspects of clinical dermatology. All academic activities are documented in a logbook and examinations are conducted yearly. Residents can proceed to the next year provided each end-of-year examination is passed with a minimum of 70%. The final exit written and practical examination is conducted at the end of the third year. Practical assessments use validated instruments, such as the Mini–Clinical Evaluation Exercise. This tool evaluates a clinical patient encounter to provide an indication of competence in skills essential for good clinical care, such as history taking, examination and clinical reasoning. The trainee receives immediate feedback to aid learning. Research methodology and a thesis are also curriculum requirements.

Kenya

Kenya is the seventh most populous country in Africa and has the third highest population in East Africa, at 53.8 million. Kenyan doctors are trained for a year in the United Kingdom, attaining a postgraduate diploma to enable them to practice in Africa. Currently, there are 30 dermatologists practicing in Kenya. The new MMed in dermatology at Moi University is the first local dermatology postgraduate training program in Kenya. The curriculum plan includes Part 1 and Part 2 examinations and a research component. Recruitment is planned to begin in 2020.

Madagascar

Madagascar has a population of 27.7 million, with 13 dermatologists. The University of Antananarivo training program includes 8 semesters of dermatology residency after completion of a basic MD degree. The 4-year program, which started in 2000 is based on the French dermatology course, Le Collège des Enseignants en Dermatologie de France (CEDEF). The curriculum was adapted for the University of Antananarivo. An evaluation needs to be passed annually in order to proceed to the next year of study. A thesis (clinical research), at least 1 scientific publication in an indexed journal (national or international journal)/semester, and participation in national and international conferences are also required.

Sudan

Sudan is the third largest country in Africa and has a population of 43.8 million, with 300 dermatologists. A dermatology training program was established in 1995 as part of the Sudan Medical Specialization Board. It started as a fellowship and later was upgraded to a 4-year master's MD program. Entry requires the candidates pass the first part examination composed of general and dermatology basic sciences plus some basic clinical dermatology. A short period of clinical training in a dermatology unit is also required. Successful candidates are enrolled in a rotational training program for the next 4 years, which includes all forms of training activities, lectures, tutorials, clinical rounds, and other specialized courses according to the curriculum. A research thesis is part of the training program. At the end of the training, a final clinical examination is conducted with the attendance of an external examiner from a recognized university. Further training opportunities include 1-year university diplomas in laser applications in medicine and general andrology. More than 500 dermatologists have graduated from the program, but some have left to practice outside of Sudan.

Tanzania

Tanzania is the fifth most populated country in Africa, with a population of 59.7 million. Dermatology care is provided by 74 dermato-venereology diplomats and 21 dermatologists. The Regional Dermatology Training Centre (RDTC) based in Moshi,[7] was established in 1992, offering a 2-year dermato-venereology course for medical assistants and clinical officers who graduate from Muhimbili University with an Advanced Diploma in Dermatovenereology. The course covers practical clinical expertise in all the major skin diseases in inpatient and outpatient settings, their public health implications, sexual health problems, and leprosy. A summative assessment, 4 written theory examinations, and 2 clinical examinations are undertaken over the 2 years. In addition, health service research projects undertaken during their only annual vacation to home communities provide a unique insight into prevalence, need, and demand for health care at the community level. A total of 290 candidates have graduated from 16 countries, 74 of whom provide service in Tanzania.

These graduates provide the backbone of dermatology services in most of sub-Saharan Africa. The graduates from all over the continent have their own society, the African Dermatovenereology Officers Association, that is recognized and has representation in the International League of Dermatological Societies (ILDS).

A 4-year MMed residency program started in 1998 and has trained 37 dermato-venereologists from sub-Saharan Africa, 19 of whom provide service in Tanzania. The residents keep supervised logbooks of all academic activities. Examinations are set by the RDTC and Tumaini University to include both theory and a practical at the end of each year for the first 2 years. A thesis with an oral defense is evaluated at the end of the third year by external examiners. This must be passed to proceed to the fourth and final year. The final examination at the end of the fourth year has written, clinical, and oral elements conducted with an external examiner. Dermatosurgery is actively taught as part of the MMed with input from plastic surgeons from abroad.

Uganda
Uganda has a population of 45.7 million, with 13 dermatologists. The Mbarara University of Science and Technology provides a 3-year dermatology residency program, which is the only training program for the country. The training involves documentation of activities in a logbook and a research component. There are 2 semesters each year with written, clinical, and oral examinations at the end of each semester. Research is presented at the end of the third year of training and an exit examination must be passed in order to graduate. Since the program's inception, 13 residents have completed training and 11 are currently enrolled.

Central Africa

The countries of Central Africa are Burundi, Cameroon, Central African Republic, Chad, Democratic Republic of the Congo, Equatorial Guinea, Gabon, São Tomé and Príncipe, and Republic of Congo Brazzaville.

The authors have been able to establish details of training only for the Democratic Republic of the Congo (**Box 5**).

The Democratic Republic of Congo
The Democratic Republic of the Congo has a population of 89.6 million. It is the fourth most populous country on the continent, is the second largest by land mass, and has 22 dermatologists. The only dermatology training program is at the University of Kinshasa, with an internship at the

---

Box 5
Key facts for Central Africa
• Dermatologist/million country inhabitants varies from 0.1 to 5.5 (see **Figs. 1** and **2**).
• One training program offered by the University of Kinshasa is in the Democratic Republic of the Congo.

University of Kinshasa Training Hospital. The training time is 5 years followed by an exit examination.

DISCUSSION
Burden of Skin Disease on the Continent

Disease burden is estimated using the disability-adjusted life year (DALY), which is a measure of health loss considering both nonfatal and fatal health burden.

The Global Burden of Disease (GBD) project provides disability and mortality data for diseases, injuries, and their risk factors stratified by age, sex, location, and time.

Data have been, and still are, collected for the GBD project from most African countries, yet secondary analysis for Africa and individual African countries is scarce.

A secondary analysis of the GBD 2017 data, explored the change in DALYs per 100,000 people over the period 1990 to 2016, and compared Botswana's burden (middle-income country) to global, high-income countries and sub-Saharan Africa burdens. Botswana's years lived with disabilities (YLDs) increased from 1990 to 2010 compared with sub-Saharan Africa, where a slow decline in the rate of YLDs over the same period was noted. In contrast, globally and in high socio-economic countries, there was a slow and constant, year-on-year increase in the rate of YLDs. Skin and subcutaneous diseases was one of the top 5 groups contributing to this increase.[8]

Current health systems in Africa respond to the causes of death but not to the long-term effects of health conditions and the associated increase in functional limitations and their effects on the health and social systems of countries. Little attention is paid to how decreased mortality relates to morbidity. The analysis of the GBD data has shown that skin and subcutaneous disease contribute to nonfatal disease burden, yet they have received little provision in health planning and financing in African countries. Dermato-venereologists per million population is abysmal despite specialist programs in the region. Considering the financial situations of many countries in

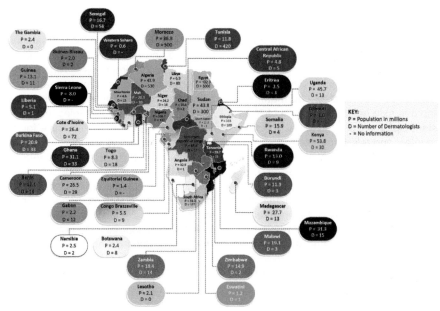

Fig. 1. Map of Africa showing *population of countries and number of dermatologists. Island states of of Cabo Verde, Comoros, Mauritius, Sao Tomé and Principe, and Seychelles are not shown. * From WorldoMeter. African Countries by population (2020). https://www.worldometers.info/population/countries-in-africa-by-population/.

Africa, where debt repayments exceed health budgets,[9] this is can be expected and will need significant lobbying to improve skin health on the continent.

Dermato-venereology Training Programs and Educational Tools on the Continent

There is limited published information on the dermato-venereology training programs in Africa.

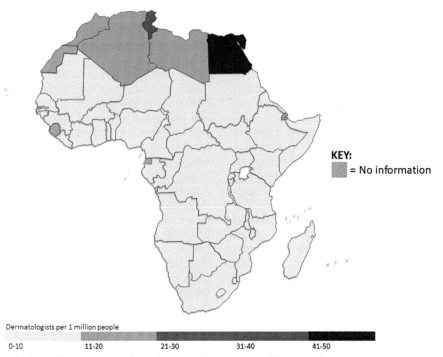

Fig. 2. Map of Africa illustrating number of dermatologists per million population.

Details from university Web sites were sparse to nonexistent at the time of this publication, making this informal survey timely. Previous attempts to highlight dermatology training in Africa focused predominantly on anglophone countries and noted that specialist training was limited. The authors discussed alternate methods of dermatology training to improve skin health delivery, including clinical assistant diplomas, short courses for generalists and nurses, and teledermatology.[4]

What is evident is that knowledge generated in high-income countries defines practices and informs thinking to the detriment of knowledge systems in African countries. Most curricula are adaptations from colonial times or taken directly from the high-income countries. Little effort has been given to the acknowledgment of local customs and knowledge to make them locally relevant and sustainable. There has been no attempt to assess the taught curricula on the continent, their origins, and relevance to local conditions despite a growing call from the younger generation on the African continent to decolonize curricula.

Calls for the decolonization of global health education and acknowledgment of the legacy of former colonial relationships and their influence on global health initiatives are increasing. Academic outputs from high-income countries dominate the global knowledge space to the point of destroying other knowledge systems (epistemicide). The balance of power mostly rests with high-income country practitioners, researchers, and scholars who set the metrics for success to their benefit and to the detriment of low-income to middle-income country knowledge systems.[10]

The educational materials available for African training programs are driven predominantly by those published in Europe, America, and the United Kingdom. The applicability of this material to those with pigmented skin in different global regions and the ability of a dermatologists, let alone a primary care health care worker, to diagnose and manage skin disorders in people of color has not been evaluated. In 2006, Ebede and Papier[18] undertook a survey of educational material dealing with pigmented skin in the United States of America. The dermatology textbooks they evaluated contained low percentages of images and textual content focused on ethnic skin: Bolognia, 19%;[11] Freedberg, 15%;[12] Rook, 12%;[13] Fitzpatrick 5th, 11%;[14] Fitzpatrick 4th, 10%;[15] Sauer, 9%;[16] and Habif, 4%.[17] From 1996 to 2005, the percentage of teaching events at the American Academy of Dermatology annual meetings that focused on skin of color has remained static at 2%. They recommended that more photographic coverage and textual information describing common and serious skin diseases in people of color should be incorporated into educational resources.[18] This highlights the inadequate educational material currently preferred and recommended for African residents.

Most training programs in Africa concentrate on modern biomedical treatment methods. Texts and guidelines written for the high-income countries emphasize the latest therapies, many of which are unavailable and not cost-effective for much of Africa. These texts give insufficient detailed information about low-technology and low-cost therapies, such as how to use honey for wound healing.[5] Additionally, the evidence base used reflects practices in high-income countries, because English studies and text are selected, and relevant studies, published in local journals, are not included by search strategies, which do not include databases, such as African Journals OnLine.[19]

Many Africans prefer consulting traditional healers who often are more accessible and affordable and are viewed as culturally appropriate. Traditional medicines are affordable, often sustainable, and locally available, for example, honey. The value of incorporating traditional medicine into training programs and curricula in African countries should be considered.[5]

There is a need for the development of programs that provide education and resources that are culturally, ethnically, and geographically appropriate. Traditional medicine practices and inexpensive, novel high-technology and low-technology educational resources that can be widely distributed and combined with telemedicine and distance learning, where appropriate, should be integrated into management options of programs.[5]

The current resurgence and interest in global health (previously termed, tropical medicine and infectious diseases and then international health) has led to the growth of partnerships, providing high-income countries with teaching and research facilities on the African continent. The article by Mbaye and colleagues[20] is timely and sobering. These investigators undertook independent PubMed searches for clinical trials and epidemiologic studies done in Africa reporting on human immunodeficiency virus and malaria (2013–2016), tuberculosis (2014–2016), salmonellosis, Ebola hemorrhagic fever, and Buruli ulcer disease (1980–2016). Of 2871 retrieved articles, 1182 were included if at least 1 laboratory test performed on biological samples had been done. Of these, 1109 (93.2%) had at least 1 Africa-based author, 552 (49.8%) had an African first author, and 41.3% (n = 458) an African last author and representation varied per diseases and study type. They report that the African continent produces only approximately 1% of the world's research publications and 0.1% of global patents.[20] The results confirmed that African researchers (particularly from nonanglophone countries) are under-represented in the most important positions (first and last authorship positions) on articles from research performed in Africa. This calls for greater investment in capacity building, incorporating practical clinical research training into residency programs, and equitable research partnerships at every level of the global health community.

Alternate programs for increasing dermato-venereology knowledge and service provision involves task shifting. The basic management of common skin diseases in French-speaking Mali is provided by 1-day training programs for primary health care workers.[21] In Western Kenya, community health workers were trained to identify and treat common dermatoses in an annual program of on-the-spot training with a dermatologist as well as a 1-weekend seminar.[22] An annual 2-month short course (with the option of upgrading to a full 1-year diploma) on basic dermatology diagnosis and management for nurses from sub-Saharan Africa was started in 1997 as a university-based combined dermatology nursing program. By 2011, 153 students had graduated who provide skin care throughout the region.[23–26] In 2011, the short course was augmented by the introduction of a university based 1-year diploma in dermatology nursing.[25] The university based 2-year diploma in dermato-venereology of the

RDTC has graduated 290 clinical assistants from sub-Saharan Africa since 1992, who are the backbone of skin care services in the region.[27]

Teledermatology can serve only as an adjunct service to sustainable dermatologic education and care in Africa.[28–30] Providing remote teledermatology services is helpful for individual difficult cases but will be insufficient to fill the global need for dermatologic care unless associated with an educational component.[29,31]

International Positioning of Africa

Only Algerian, Angolan, Mauritian, South African, Libyan, Moroccan, Nigerian, Tunisian, and 3 Egyptian societies are members of the ILDS, according to their Web site.[31] The new African Society of Dermatology and Venerology (representing dermatologists in sub-Saharan Africa), African Dermato-venereology Officers Association (representing dermato-venereology diplomats in sub-Saharan Africa), and francophone African Society of Dermatology are also members. The African Association for Dermatology still has membership status although it no longer operates per its constitution and thus is not representative of Africa.[32]

Most drug trials and clinical studies on which guidelines and management options are based exclude participants from Africa, do not include participants of various race and ethnicity, or, if included, do not interpret results accordingly. Kaufman and colleagues[33] investigated these issues by analyzing atopic dermatitis clinical trials published

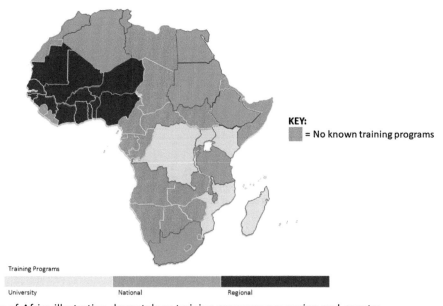

KEY:
= No known training programs

Training Programs

University   National   Regional

Fig. 3. Map of Africa illustrating dermatology training programs per region and country.

Table 1
General information on dermatology per region and country in Africa

Region	Country	Dermatology Society	Population (in Millions)[a]	Dermatologists	Dermatology Training Program Regional or National	Dermatology Training Program University
West Africa	Benin	Yes	12.1	18	Regional	No
	Burkina Faso	Yes	20.9	33	Regional	No
	Cabo Verde	—	0.6	—	—	—
	Côte d'Ivoire	Yes	26.4	72	Regional	No
	The Gambia	No	2.4	0	No	No
	Ghana	Yes	31.1	33	Regional	Yes
	Guinea Conakry	Yes	13.1	11	Regional	Yes
	Guinea-Bissau	No	2.0	2	Regional	No
	Liberia	—	5.1	1	—	—
	Mali	Yes	20.3	30	Regional	No
	Niger	Yes	24.2	16	No	No
	Nigeria	Yes	206.1	132	Regional	Yes
	Senegal	Yes	16.7	54	Regional	Yes
	Sierra Leone	—	8	—	—	—
	Togo	Yes	8.3	18	Regional	Yes
East Africa	Comoros	—	0.9	—	—	—
	Djibouti	—	1	—	—	—
	Eritrea	No	3.5	1	No	No
	Ethiopia	Yes	115	100	National	Yes
	Kenya	Yes	53.8	30	No	Yes
	Madagascar	Yes	27.7	13	No	Yes
	Mauritius	—	1.3	—	—	—
	Rwanda	Yes	13	9	No	No
	Seychelles	—	0.1	—	—	—
	Somalia	No	15.9	4	No	No
	South Sudan	—	11.2	1	—	—
	Sudan	Yes	43.8	300	National	Yes
	Tanzania	Yes	59.7	21	National	Yes
	Uganda	No	45.7	13	No	Yes

Region	Country					
North Africa	Algeria	Yes	43.9	National	530	Yes
	Egypt	Yes	102.3	National	5000	Yes
	Libya	Yes	6.9	National	80	Yes
	Mauritania	Yes	4.6	No	15	No
	Morocco	Yes	36.9	National	500	Yes
	Sahrawi Arab Democratic Republic (Western Sahara)	—	0.6	—	—	—
	Tunisia	Yes	11.8	National	420	Yes
Central Africa	Burundi	No	11.9	No	3	No
	Cameroon	Yes	26.5	No	29	No
	Central African Republic	No	4.8	No	5	No
	Chad	No	16.4	No	2	No
	Congo Republic Brazzaville	Yes	5.5	No	9	No
	Democratic Republic of the Congo	Yes	89.6	No	22	Yes
	Equatorial Guinea	—	1.4	—	—	—
	Gabon	Yes	2.2	No	12	No
	São Tomé and Príncipe	—	0.2	—	—	—
Southern Africa	Angola	Yes	32.9	No	1	No
	Botswana	No	2.4	No	8	No
	Eswatini	No	1.2	No	1	No
	Lesotho	No	2.1	No	0	No
	Malawi	Yes	19.1	No	3	No
	Mozambique	No	31.3	No	15	Yes
	Namibia	No	2.5	No	2	No
	South Africa	Yes	59.3	National	177	No
	Zambia	No	18.4	No	14	No
	Zimbabwe	No	14.9	No	2	No

—, Data not available at the time of publication.
[a] https://www.worldometers.info/population/countries-in-africa-by-population/.
Data From WorldoMeter. Contries in Africa by population. African Countries by population (2020). https://www.worldometers.info/population/countries-in-africa-by-population/

Table 2
Summary of training programs and curricula in Africa

Region	Country	Dermatology Specialization Qualification	Length (in Years)	Exit Examination	Additional Training	Thesis	Portfolio	Entry Requirements First Professional Qualification and Additional Expertise
West Africa	Benin	aYes	4	Yes	No	Yes	Yes	MD or specialty Internship
	Burkina Faso	Diploma (DES Dermatologie)	4	Yes	No	Yes	Yes	MD or specialty Internship
	Côte d'Ivoire	Diploma (DES Dermatologie)	4	Yes	No	No	No	Diploma of General Practitioner
	Ghana	Fellowship (Fellowship of the West African College of Physicians or the Fellowship of the Ghana College of Physicians and Surgeons)	5 (3 in dermatology)	Yes	No	Yes	Yes	MBChB, after part 1 of internal medicine
	Guinea Conakry	aYes	4	Yes	No	Yes	Yes	bFPQ
	Mali	aYes	4	Yes	No	Yes	Yes	MD or specialty Internship
	Nigeria	Fellowship Internal Medicine subspecialty Dermatology	5 (3 in dermatology)	Yes	No	Yes	Yes	MBBS/MBChB and after Part 1 in internal medicine
	Senegal	Diploma (Specialist in Dermatology)	4	Yes	No	Yes	Yes	MD and national residency contest
	Togo	aYes	4	Yes	No	Yes	Yes	MD or specialty Internship
East Africa	Ethiopia	Diploma (Specialty Certificate in Dermatovenereology)	3	Yes	No	Yes	Yes	MD
	Kenya	MMed	4	Yes	No	Yes	Yes	MBChB
	Madagascar	Fellowship with certificate French DEFS and AFS	4	Yes	No	Yes	No	MD and general intern examination

Region	Country	Qualification	Duration (y)		Subspecialty diplomas			Basic medical degree
	Sudan	MD	4	Yes	1-y university diplomas in laser applications in medicine and 1 in general andrology	Yes	Yes	MBBS
	Tanzania	ADDV	2	Yes	No	No	No	Clinical Assistant
		MMed	4	Yes	No	Yes	Yes	MBChB
	Uganda	MMed	3	Yes	No	Yes	Yes	MBChB, plus 1 y of full clinical practice
North Africa	Algeria	aYes	4	Yes	—	Yes	Yes	bFPQ
	Egypt	MMed	3	Yes	1-y Diploma in lasers and 1 in aesthetics	No	Yes	MBChB plus grade
		Fellowship	5	Yes		No	Yes	MBChB plus grade
		MD/PhD	5	Yes		Yes	Yes	MBChB plus grade
	Libya	MSc	2	Yes	No	Yes	No	MBChB, selection examination
		Fellowship	4	Yes	No	Yes	Yes	MBChB, selection examination
	Morocco	aYes	4	Yes	—	Yes	Yes	bFPQ
	Tunisia	Diploma (DES Dermatologie)	4	No	No	No	No	MD, Diplôme de Doctorat en Médecine, and national examination
Central Africa	Democratic Republic of the Congo	Diploma (Doctor Specialist in dermatology)	5	Yes	No	Yes	Yes	Diplome de docteur en medecine chirurgie et accouchement
Southern Africa	Mozambique	Diploma (Specialist in Dermatology and Venereology)	5 (3 in dermatology)	Yes	No	No	Yes	MD diploma, selection examination, and after Part 1 in internal medicine
	South Africa	Fellowship	4	Yes	Aesthetics, surgery	No	Yes	MBChB/MBBCh with additional experience
		MMed	4	Yes		Yes	Yes	

Abbreviations: ADDV, Advanced Diploma in Dermatovenereology; AFS, Attestation de Formation Spécialisée; DES, Diplôme d'études spécialisées; DEFS, Diplôme d'Études de Formation Spécialisée; FPQ, First Professional Qualification.

—, Data not available at the time of publication.

a Dermatology specialization available but qualification not established by the time of publication.

b First professional qualification not established by the time of publication.

Data From WorldoMeter. Contries in Africa by population. African Countries in Africa by population (2020). https://www.worldometers.info/population/countries-in-africa-by-population/

between 2000 and 2009. Most patients included were white (62.1%), followed by black (18.0%), Asian (6.9%), and Hispanic (2.0%). Only 59.5% of studies included race and ethnicity as baseline demographic information. Only 10.3% of studies commented on race or ethnicity in the interpretation of results, making it difficult to extrapolate the results to other ethnic groups. There is underrepresentation of African participants in clinical trials as well as lack of subset analyses by race.[33]

SUMMARY AND RECOMMENDATIONS

Regions that have dermatology or dermato-venereology training programs follow regional, national, or university curricula (**Fig. 3**, **Tables 1** and **2**).

> Regional program and harmonized curriculum (West Africa): anglophone—Ghana and Nigeria; francophone—Benin, Burkina Faso, Côte d'Ivoire, Guinea Conakry, Guinea-Bissau, Mali, Mauritania, Niger, Senegal, and Togo.
> National program, curriculum, and accreditation: Algeria, Egypt, Ethiopia, Morocco, Sudan, South Africa, Tanzania (RDTC), and Tunisia.
> University program, curriculum, and accreditation: Democratic Republic of the Congo, Kenya (Moi), Madagascar (Antananarivo University), Mozambique, and Uganda (Mbarara).

There is little sharing of curricula and training programs between the various universities, highlighting the need for pooling of expertise and resources so that training can be strengthened regionally and curricula developed that are relevant to local African needs.

Based on the authors' informal survey, the ratio of dermatologists to population across the continent is illustrated in **Figs. 1** and **2** and **Table 1**. Apart from the Northern region, where it ranges from 8 to 49 dermatologists per million population, the rest of the continent has fewer than 10 dermatologists per million population, usually fewer than 1 dermatologist per million population.

Continent-wide and region-wide surveys of dermatologists trained, their distribution in countries, their retention profiles, and their contributions to both undergraduate and postgraduate dermato-venereology training and curriculum decolonization should be undertaken. Also, of importance would be surveys of how this contribution of dermato-venereology to the health burden is recognized and funded throughout the continent both regarding clinical services to the population and training funding.

Continent collaboration should embrace local platforms, such as the Alliance for Accelerating Excellence in Science in Africa (AESA). Launched in 2015, AESA is an Africa-led, Africa-centered, and Africa-specific funding and agenda setting platform created to accelerate scientific excellence, leadership and innovation.[34]

One example of successful bidirectional exchange is the International Federation of Medical Students' Associations. Since the 1950s, more than 15,000 exchanges have taken place annually in more than 127 countries. This is a student-led organization; each outgoing student pays in their local currency for the cost of an incoming student and that student's cost of living.[35]

CLINICS CARE POINTS

- There is a paucity or dermatologists, <1 per million population, for most of the continent.
- Dermatology training programs are present in 25 of the 55 countries across the continent.
- Training programs are of international standard.
- Graduates are competent clinicians, knowledgeable of local customs and needs.
- Programs often reflect colonial roots and need de-colonisation making them relevant to Africa.

ACKNOWLEDGMENTS

Adebola Ogunbiyi, Abdelmajid Khelif, Amina N Ouedraogo, Ayesha O Akinkugbe, Bérénice KE Degboe, Célestin Ahogo, Christian Muteba Baseke, Daudi Mavura, Emmanuel K. Ekyinabah, Evanson Kamuri, Gamal Duweb, Garba Mahamadou, Grace Mulyowa, Fahafahantsoa Rapelanoro Rabenja, Fatimata Ly, Haji Ntaibu, Jean Marie Rukanikigitero, Kayitesi Kayitenkore, Mahira el Sayed, Maged El-Batawi, Mamadou D. Ball, Margaret Yaa Lartey, Nejib Doss, Niamba Pascal, Osman Faye, Rogers Nonde, Rolanda Manuel, Roop Saini, Safi Eldin Ali, Silvio Coelho, Tsevuru Munhutu, Workalemahu Alemu, and Wendemagegn Yeshanehe for their input on training programs. A special word of thanks goes to Ms Phakama Jika for her assistance with the manuscript graphics.

REFERENCES

1. Mwaniki A. The 10 most populated countries in Africa. World Atlas 2018. Available at: https://www.worldatlas.com/articles/the-10-most-populated-countries-in-africa.html. Accessed May 30, 2020.
2. Regions of the African Union. Available at: https://en.wikipedia.org/wiki/Regions_of_the_African_Union. Accessed June 2, 2020.
3. Epidemiology and management of common skin diseases in children in developing countries. WHO/FCH/CAH/05.12.

4. Hay RJ, Fuller LC. The assessment of dermatological needs in resource-poor regions. Int J Dermatol 2011;50(5):552–7.

5. Hu J, McKoy K, Papier A, et al. Dermatology and HIV/AIDS in Africa. J Glob Infect Dis 2011;3(3):275–80.

6. La Société Tunisienne de Dermatologie et de Vénéréologie (STDV). Available at: https://stdv.tn/college-de-dermatologie/. Accessed May 30, 2020.

7. Regional Dermatology Training Centre (RDTC). Available at: https://rdtc.go.tz/. Accessed May 30, 2020.

8. Hanass-Hancock J, Carpenter B. Trends in health and disability in Botswana. An analysis of the global burden of disease study, [published online ahead of print, 2020 Apr 1]. Disabil Rehabil 2020;1-7. https://doi.org/10.1080/09638288.2020.1743774.

9. Comparing debt payments with health spending. Jubilee Debt Campaign; 2020. Available at: https://jubileedebt.org.uk/wp-content/uploads/2020/04/Debt-payments-and-health-spending_13.04.20.pdf. Accessed May 30, 2020.

10. Eichbaum QG, Adams LV, Evert J, et al. Decolonizing global health education: rethinking institutional partnerships and approaches [published online ahead of print, 2020 Apr 28]. Acad Med 2020. https://doi.org/10.1097/ACM.0000000000003473.

11. Bolognia JL, Jorizzo JL, Rapini RP, et al, editors. Dermatology. Philadelphia: Mosby; 2003.

12. Freedberg IM, Eisen AZ, Wolff K, et al, editors. Fitzpatrick's dermatology in general medicine. 6th edition. New York: McGraw-Hill; 2003.

13. Burns T, editor. Rook's textbook of dermatology. 7th edition. Boston: Blackwell Science; 2004.

14. Wolff K, Johnson RA, Suurmond D, editors. Fitzpatrick's color atlas and synopsis of clinical dermatology. 5th edition. New York: McGraw-Hill; 2005.

15. Fitzpatrick TB, Johnson RA, Wolff K, et al, editors. Color atlas and synopsis of clinical dermatology. 4th edition. New York: McGraw-Hill; 2001.

16. Hall JC, editor. Sauer's manual of skin diseases. 8th edition. Philadelphia: Lippincott Williams and Wilkins; 2000.

17. Habif TP, editor. Clinical dermatology: a color guide to diagnosis and therapy. 4th edition. Philadelphia: Mosby; 2004.

18. Ebede T, Papier A. Disparities in dermatology educational resources. J Am Acad Dermatol 2006;55(4):687–90.

19. African Journals Online (AJOL). Available at: https://www.ajol.info/index.php/ajol. Accessed May 30, 2020.

20. Mbaye R, Gebeyehu R, Hossmann S, et al. Who is telling the story? A systematic review of authorship for infectious disease research conducted in Africa, 1980-2016. BMJ Glob Health 2019;4(5):e001855.

21. Mahé A, Faye O, N'Diaye HT, et al. Integration of basic dermatological care into primary health care services in Mali. Bull World Health Organ 2005;83(12):935–41.

22. Schmeller W. Community health workers reduce skin diseases in East African children. Int J Dermatol 1998;37(5):370–7.

23. Cloete D. Dermatology nursing in a rural area - the Overberg experience. Community dermatology in a rural area in the Western Cape. CME 2013;31(7):254–8. African Journals Online (AJOL). Available at: https://www.ajol.info/. Accessed May 30, 2020.

24. Stevens J. Dermatology nursing in the community: The Mitchells Plain experience. Dermatology is an important element of community nursing. CME 2013;31(7):250–3. African Journals Online (AJOL). Available at: https://www.ajol.info/. Accessed May 30, 2020.

25. Kelly PA. Community dermatology nursing in resource-poor communities across Africa. J Dermatol Nurses Assoc 2012;4(4):244–8.

26. Ersser SJ, Kaur V, Kelly P, et al. Community dermatology. The contribution of the nursing service worldwide and its capacity to benefit within the dermatology field. Int J Dermatol 2011;50(5):582–9.

27. Hay RJ. Regional Dermatology Training Centre in Moshi, Tanzania – pursuing a dream. Continuing Medical Education 2013;31(7):262–4. African Journals Online (AJOL). Available at: http://www.cmej.org.za/index.php/cmej/article/view/2814/3087 https://www.ajol.info/. Accessed May 30, 2020.

28. Faye O, Bagayoko CO, Dicko A, et al, Teledermali Team. A teledermatology pilot programme for the management of skin diseases in primary health care centres: Experiences from a resource-limited country (Mali, West Africa). Trop Med Infect Dis 2018;3(3):88.

29. Hay R, Estrada R, Grossmann H. Managing skin disease in resource-poor environments – the role of community-oriented training and control programs. Int J Dermatol 2011;50(5):558–63.

30. Weinberg J, Kaddu S, Gabler G, et al. The African teledermatology project: Providing access to dermatologic care and education in sub-Saharan Africa. Pan Afr Med J 2009;3:16.

31. Colven R1, Shim MH, Brock D, et al. Dermatological diagnostic acumen improves with use of a simple telemedicine system for underserved areas of South Africa. Telemed J E Health 2011;17(5):363–9.

32. International League of Dermatological Societies (ILDS). Available at: https://ilds.org/. Accessed May 30, 2020.

33. Kaufman BP, Guttman-Yassky E, Alexis AF. Atopic dermatitis in diverse racial and ethnic groups -Variations in epidemiology, genetics, clinical presentation and treatment. Exp Dermatol 2018;27(4):340–57.

34. Alliance for Accelerating Excellence in Science in Africa (AESA). Available at: https://www.aasciences.africa/aesa. Accessed May 30, 2020.

35. International Federation of Medical Student Associations (IFMSA). Available at: https://ifmsa.org/professional-exchanges/. Accessed May 30, 2020.

Developing a Platform for Global Health Dermatology Mentorship and Collaboration

Introducing the International Alliance for Global Health Dermatology

Linda Oyesiku, MPH[a,b], Devon E. McMahon, BA[b],
Lucinda Claire Fuller, MA, RFCP[c,d], Esther E. Freeman, MD, PhD[a,*]

KEYWORDS

- Dermatology • Dermatopathology • Neglected tropical diseases • Global health • Teledermatology
- Mentorship • Medical education • Volunteerism

KEY POINTS

- The International Alliance for Global Health Dermatology (GLODERM) was founded in 2019.
- GLODERM aims to fill a critical gap in providing key resources, mentorship opportunities, and exposure to the breadth of the field of global health in the context of dermatology.
- GLODERM will place a significant focus on advocacy and policy to be prioritized in global health dermatology to achieve the international vision of dermatology.

INTRODUCTION

Dermatology has an important place in the global health agenda. Skin disease is the fourth leading cause of nonfatal disease burden in both disability adjusted life years and years lost to disability worldwide.[1,2] There is enormous potential for interventions in public health dermatology to lessen skin disease burden and narrow gaps in access to care.[3,4]

Like global health tracks in other medical specialties, global health dermatology is rapidly expanding in medical education, telehealth, capacity building, task shifting, research, and academic career development.[5–11] In the United States, medical school education and postgraduate residency programs in dermatology have responded to this growing interest by developing or expanding opportunities for dermatologists to develop a skillset in global health.[5,12] In the United Kingdom, the British Association of Dermatologists have established a Global Health Dermatology focus to share best practice in global health dermatology. Despite this growing interest, there is still a shortage of dermatologists worldwide, particularly in countries where the burden of skin diseases is greatest.[13] To this end, numerous efforts are under way to increase access to dermatology training[5] and both build capacity and "task shift"[14] to close this gap in access to care and treatment.[13]

Main priorities in global health dermatology include funding for research and increased focus on advocacy and policy development.[2,4]

[a] University of Miami Miller School of Medicine, Miami, FL, USA; [b] Department of Dermatology, Massachusetts General Hospital, Harvard Medical School, Boston, MA, USA; [c] International Foundation for Dermatology, Willan House, 4 Fitzroy Square, London W1T 5HQ, UK; [d] Chelsea and Westminster Hospital NHS Foundation Trust, 369 Fulham Road, London SW10 9NH, UK
* Corresponding author. 50 Staniford Street, Boston, MA 02114.
E-mail address: efreeman@mgh.harvard.edu

Dermatol Clin 39 (2021) 73–82
https://doi.org/10.1016/j.det.2020.08.007

From an advocacy standpoint, the inclusion of dermatologic medications in the World Health Organization (WHO) List of Essential Medicines was pivotal to acknowledging the importance of skin health and treating disfiguring and stigmatizing skin diseases that affect vulnerable populations worldwide.[2] Dermatologists in the International Alliance for the Control of Scabies (IACS) contributed to establishing scabies as an official Neglected Tropical Disease (NTD) by WHO and the addition of ivermectin to the WHO list of essential medicines to treat ectoparasitic infections.[15,16] These inclusions signaled a powerful acknowledgment that dermatologic conditions are a public health priority and started the move toward creating an integrated approach to addressing skin NTDs on a global scale.[6,8] WHO has published guidelines, epidemiologic reports, and training guides on skin conditions in addition to establishing a dedicated skin NTD Web site to assist providers in the diagnosis and treatment of skin diseases.[17-19] These guidelines emerged from growing requests from providers around the world in need of guidance to address the skin health needs in their communities. Other areas of increasing attention and significant impact include refugee/migrant dermatology and climate change dermatology.[20,21]

The aim of this article was to highlight a selection of current organizations; discuss existing opportunities and identify areas of need in global health dermatology; describe the development of a new international alliance; propose future directions; and reflect on lessons learned.

THE NEED FOR AN OPEN GLOBAL ALLIANCE
Key Components of a Global Alliance

The International League of Dermatologic Societies (ILDS) Grand Challenges exercise concluded that to achieve global skin health there are 4 key measures: (1) research, (2) education, (3) clinical application through translation, and (4) support of those responsible in the management and delivery of health care at local and national levels.[22] Previously, an alliance aiming to unite efforts toward skin health that was open to international participation from colleagues at any stage of training or profession, from physicians to industry, to pharmacists and epidemiologists was lacking. A number of organizations and key stakeholders developed foundations, subcommittees, exchanges, and disease-specific alliances to address each individual measure, but none all encompassing (**Table 1**).

We have since called for the field of dermatology to assert its presence on the global stage[6] with strategies that echo the key measures of ILDS[22]: (1) develop champions to advance dermatologic initiatives within health policy organizations at both national and international levels, (2) pursue quality research with an international and epidemiologic focus, and (3) expand the role of global health in the education of our dermatology trainees across the world. A global alliance could serve as a task force for organizing these efforts uniting under one voice and providing a home for the expansion of an effective global health dermatology community.

The aim of the alliance is to address these calls for an entity in which individuals and partners dedicated to global health dermatology can find community and collaboration. It will work on delineating career models for trainees; providing advocacy through research, and establishing a strong united voice for the field of dermatology on the global health stage.[4,23] The alliance provides a potential cohort of experts to work with international health agencies to facilitate the creation of standardized data recording and assessment of the global burden of skin disease, fueling efforts to improve skin health globally.[2,23] The alliance intends to harmonize research and implementation programs by addressing community-defined gaps in research while coordinating the expertise of multiple individuals and partners with the same goal.

The Need for Training and Mentorship

For trainees in dermatology with an interest in global health, the opportunity to follow a well-defined career path in global health dermatology is important for confidence in choosing the specialty and finding mentors to guide their progress. For mentors, identifying mentees is essential for establishing future generations of global health dermatologists and effective succession. Organizations and alliances serve as potential launching pads for trainees, connecting them with funding opportunities, research experiences, and mentors.

Graduate medical training opportunities for global health dermatology are scanty, although a few well-established opportunities exist, such as The American Academy of Dermatology Resident International Grant and the Native American Health Service resident rotations.[9,12,24] GLODERM seeks to provide a forum to support graduates of programs such as these to share knowledge with the next generation of trainees. Adequate preparation and mentorship are particularly important in global health work during

Table 1
Examples of global health dermatology organizations and alliances

Name of Organization	Founded	Membership	Mission	Scope of Work
International Society of Dermatology (ISD)	1959	Any dermatologist, resident medical student, fellow or scientist interested in dermatology	To offer excellence in education, mentorship, and networking for the global dermatology community through meetings, communications, and promotion of professionalism and diversity to improve patient care.[31]	Global dermatology, tropical skin diseases, venereology, climate change, and public health, and teaching dermatology in developing countries.
International Foundation of Dermatology (IFD)	1987	Dermatology organizations (not individuals)	To increase awareness, cooperation, and communication within the global dermatology community to promote high-quality education, clinical care, research, and innovation that will improve skin health globally.[32]	Humanitarian arm of the International League of Dermatologic Societies (ILDS).
Regional Dermatology Training Center (RDTC)	1990	Trained consultants, medical assistants, and clinical officers	Created as a space meant to train and build capacity in East Africa. Supra-regional training, research and clinical center. It provides care to dermatologic patients and training to medical assistants and clinical officers.[33] RDTC has trained 290 graduates from 17 countries. The MMed Residents Program has trained 37 Consultants from 7 African countries.	Established in partnership with the IFD, Tanzanian Ministry of Health and Kilimanjaro Christian Medical Center (KCMC). It is also home to the Care Unit for Persons with Albinism (CUPWA) at RDTC Tanzania. Recognized by the World Health Organization as a training center for skin disease, leprosy, and sexually transmitted infections.

(continued on next page)

Table 1
(continued)

Name of Organization	Founded	Membership	Mission	Scope of Work
Dermatología Comunitaria	1991	Trained Dermatologists	A reference center for teaching and research on tropical neglected diseases in Latin America, an important center of teledermatology and to produce quality research.[34]	Community Dermatology as a phrase was coined by a group in Mexico to describe applying a health care system to help manage the burden of skin disease on a community level with an understanding of local health needs.[35] It became a subspecialty with a focus on epidemiology and public health using needs-assessments to address gaps in care and treat a community's most common skin diseases.
International Society of Dermatology in the Tropics	1996	Doctors, scientists, medical nursing, and auxiliary staff	To promote adequate and qualified dermatologic care for the population living in tropical and subtropical countries.[36]	The society offers seminars for a certificate of travel and tropical dermatology.
International Alliance for Control of Scabies (IACS)	2012	Researchers, clinicians, and public health experts	A global network committed to the control of human scabies and the promotion of health and well-being of all those living in affected communities.[37]	Facilitated the development of global priorities for control and surveillance and global diagnostic criteria for scabies.[38]
International Alliance for Global Health Dermatology (GLODERM)	2019	Any individual interested in dermatology	Our mission is to promote skin health worldwide through enhanced access to care, training, advocacy, capacity building, clinical care, and research.	We aim to raise awareness about skin health within the overall well-being of communities and to reduce the burden of both common and neglected skin diseases.

training.[7,25,26] A significant gap in global health career development is the creation of avenues for mentors to have access to trainees and acknowledging a mentor's contribution to trainees with support, whether through dedicated time or funding.[11]

One of the goals of GLODERM is to create an environment to support trainees from all over the world interested in global health dermatology and share and develop potential career models. The hope is that the alliance will fill a critical gap in providing key resources, mentorship opportunities, and general exposure to the breadth of the field of global health in the context of dermatology.

THE FOUNDING OF THE INTERNATIONAL ALLIANCE FOR GLOBAL HEALTH DERMATOLOGY

After several years of discussion among global health dermatology experts at various international meetings, a small group of dermatologists created a steering group to bring the idea of a truly open access alliance of global dermatology to fruition. The group met at the Association for Tropical Medicine and Hygiene 2018 annual meeting and set about mapping the next steps to progress for the establishment of a global health dermatology alliance, and GLODERM (the International Alliance of Global Health Dermatology) was born.

At the AAD 2019, GLODERM had its first annual meeting with an academic symposium and business meeting. More than 60 international participants learned about the goals of the alliance and the breadth of the subspecialty, and were invited to join this new group. The symposium included talks on teledermatology in resource-poor settings, community dermatology, institutional partnerships, advocacy in international organizations, and refugee and migrant dermatology. A mentorship in global health panel was held to share insight and guidance on finding and working with mentors to establish a career path, how to gain research and clinical experience as a trainee, and finding work-life balance.

A vision and mission statement emerged from the meeting:

Vision statement: Skin health for everyone, everywhere.

Mission statement: We envision a world where every individual, regardless of background, has the opportunity to achieve skin health. Our mission is to promote skin health worldwide through enhanced access to care, training, advocacy, capacity building, clinical care, and research. We aim to raise awareness about skin health within the overall well-being of communities and to reduce the burden of both common and neglected skin diseases.

Forging an Identity

The development of a logo (**Fig. 1**) and a digital presence in the form of a Web site (gloderm.org) was critical to the launch of GLODERM and building a membership base that tripled in the first 6 months of its founding. The Web site (**Fig. 2**) has attracted visitors from 87 countries (**Fig. 3**). One of the key roles of the Web site is to serve as a repository for research publications in global health dermatology, training opportunities, and a project map of areas where GLODERM members work and collaborate. These components are central to the mission of GLODERM providing a platform for collaboration and information.

The training resources page currently serves as a list of opportunities in global health dermatology. A global health dermatology roadmap and a panel of mentors is in development to provide interested trainees affirmation and validation for the potential path ahead, as well as show the prospects for the diverse career models. For trainees, these opportunities may reinforce their decision to pursue global health dermatology by allowing exposure to this field early on in their careers.

Organizational Partners

Building alliances with other organizations involved in global health dermatology is important for the effectiveness of GLODERM. Gaining support from the International Foundation of Dermatology (IFD) has been particularly critical, as the IFD has agreed to assist with organizational development and secretariat support. Being accepted as a member of the Neglected Tropical Diseases Nongovernmental Organization Network has put GLODERM on the map in the context of International Health Agency recognition with the WHO.

GL⊕DERM

International Alliance for Global Health Dermatology

Fig. 1. GLODERM logo and logotype.

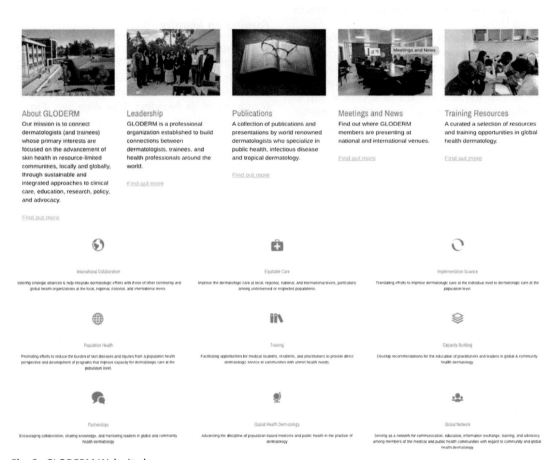

Fig. 2. GLODERM Web site home page.

The International Society of Dermatology has provided key annual meeting financial and administrative support and undertakes to promote the cause. The IACS, which has just embarked on a World Scabies Elimination Program, benefits from collaboration and shares many members with GLODERM. These cross-cutting partnerships increase the potential for collaboration and support across organizations.

Social Media

Social media is an additional realm for GLODERM (@glodermalliance) to carry out its mission. Social media has become increasingly popular as a platform to educate the public, raise awareness, and collaborate with colleagues in the field of dermatology.[27] GLODERM stands to benefit from a social media presence, particularly for the recruitment of members and increased visibility. Each social media platform has unique potential based on its format (**Box 1**).

Mentorship

A key area for GLODERM's impact is the creation of a space in which trainees can evaluate a potential career path and nourish their interest by connecting with practicing dermatologists in the field of global health dermatology. Although the specialty of dermatology is relatively small, the number of global health dermatologists is even smaller. Networking is an essential component in professional development in general, but it is particularly critical when trainees are at institutions where they cannot identify a global health mentor in their department or their country. The scarcity of dermatologists in some countries and

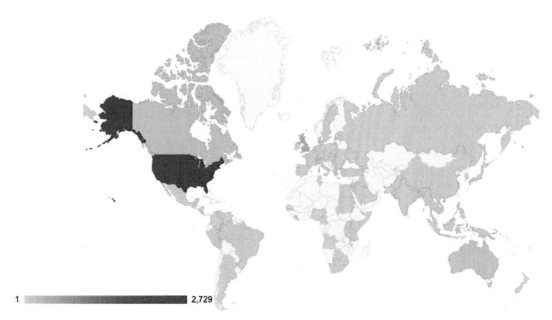

Fig. 3. GLODERM Web site traffic since February 2019. The Web site has attracted 2729 visitors from 87 countries.

particularly dermatology research mentors is well documented; this too could severely limit career potential and cause interests to wane due to lack of human resources.[28,29] GLODERM strives to serve as an alliance to connect health professionals in various stages of their career with global health dermatology mentors. These relationships can help facilitate advanced training opportunities, and research and teaching opportunities, laying the groundwork for a more impactful and longitudinal career in global health.

Box 1
International Alliance for Global Health Dermatology use of social media

Instagram @glodermalliance

    Broad crowd-sourcing potential

    Educational Platform

Twitter @glodermalliance

    Global community engagement

    Attracting support and recruiting new members

    Educational platform

Other digital media

    Dialogues in Dermatology Podcast

    Journal of Investigative Dermatology Podcast

Ethics

Last, GLODERM strives to equip trainees and practitioners with a sound understanding of the ethical dimensions of global health and the challenges of cultural competency and sensitivity. There are existing privileges that often afford opportunities and benefits to trainees in higher income countries to work overseas compared with the relative scarcity of opportunity for trainees in low-income and middle-income countries, resulting in an uneven exchange that is sometimes not mutually beneficial.[9,29,30] With a keen awareness and commitment to mutual advantage, GLODERM intends to be inclusive, recognizing that true collaboration and alliance in global health dermatology must be a two-way transaction.

FUTURE DIRECTIONS FOR THE INTERNATIONAL ALLIANCE FOR GLOBAL HEALTH DERMATOLOGY

Now in its second year, GLODERM continues to grow, adapt, and respond to the needs of its members and the communities that members serve locally and globally, as well as build opportunities for research and mentorship for trainees. GLODERM has 6 areas of focus for the future: (1) expanding leadership and membership diversity; (2) subspecialty expertise taskforce or working group development to address specific areas for mentorship, advocacy, and research; (3) increasing output of epidemiologic representative

<table>
<tr><td>

Box 2
Future directions for International Alliance for Global Health Dermatology (GLODERM)

Global Leadership Diversity

- Electing regional members to the advisory board and steering committee
- Building a collaborative space for creating global priorities in reducing the global burden of skin disease
- Advocacy for inclusion of skin diseases in global health organizations

Subject area expertise Web pages on gloderm. org

- Database of subject area experts open to serve as mentors
- Establishing a starting point for planning research and publications
- Creation of working groups or taskforces
  - Curating a collection of and developing manuals with best practice and treatment algorithms

Representative data and epidemiologic research

- A forum for rigorous standardization of data recording AND diagnostic criteria to demonstrate the burden and implement strategies for increasing access to high quality care.
- Research will allow us to implement strategies for increasing access to high-quality care

Ethical issues in researching, teaching, and practicing abroad

- Developing a GLODERM Best Practices Guide in global health dermatology

Cultivating relationships with other associations and alliances

- Establishing a presence at other annual meetings in dermatology for rotating regional GLODERM annual meetings

Expanding a social media presence

- Advertising opportunities and informal global engagement
- Instagram @glodermalliance
  - Broad crowd-sourcing potential
  - Educational platform
  - Showcasing careers in global health to trainees
- Twitter @glodermalliance
  - Increasing global community engagement
  - Attracting support and recruiting new members

</td></tr>
</table>

○ Using the educational platform and the growing influence of #dermtwitter

data; (4) discussing issues surrounding ethics of researching, teaching, training, and practicing internationally; (5) establishing GLODERM's presence at regional annual meetings; and (6) expanding GLODERM's social media presence (**Box 2**).

SUMMARY

There is a clear and urgent need for collaboration, mentorship, and capacity building in global health dermatology. In addition, champions are required to advocate for quality funding for research. Highlighting the work of global health dermatologists is important in increasing the visibility of the subspecialty for the multitude of reasons mentioned in this article. GLODERM intends to be a space in which people can find information on funding, fellowship, and mentorship opportunities. Last, to continue to grow as a truly global alliance, GLODERM needs to increase involvement from low-income and middle-income countries. It plans to achieve this with targeted advocacy, scheduling future GLODERM meetings alongside significant international dermatology conferences such as the African Society of Dermatology and Venereology meeting, the European Academy of Dermatology (EADV) meeting (Vienna 2020) and International Congress of Dermatology (Melbourne November 2021) World Congress of Dermatology meeting.

The founding and launch at the American Academy of Dermatology (AAD) 2019 annual meeting of the International Alliance for Global Health Dermatology (GLODERM), as a new entity to unite dermatologists, allied health professionals, and trainees was a pivotal moment. It began as a group of 12 people that grew to 60 members at the inaugural meeting in 2019. Over the past year, membership has grown to 235 dermatologists, nurses, trainees, and public health professionals from all over the world working toward achieving the international vision of dermatology; skin health for everyone, everywhere.

ACKNOWLEDGMENTS

The authors gratefully acknowledge Erin Amerson, MD; Justin Bandino, MD; Helmut Beltraminelli, MD; Kimberly Breglio, MD, PhD; Isabel Casas, MD; Aileen Chang, MD; Olivier Chosidow, MD, PhD; Sarah Coates, MD; Ousmane Faye, MD, PhD; Amy Forrestel, MD; Roderick Hay, MD; Alexia Knapp, MD, MS; Carrie Kovarik, MD; Toby

Maurer, MD; Scott Norton, MD, MPH, MSc; Wingfield Rehmus, MD, MPH; Colette Van Hees, MD; Karolyn Wanat, MD; Margot Whitfield, MD; Victoria Williams, MD; and Nicholas Schenck-Smith, BS, for their consult and contributions to the founding of GLODERM.

DISCLOSURE

E.E. Freeman is supported by an NIH Career Development Award K23AI36579. L.C. Fuller is Chair of the International Foundation for Dermatology. L. Oyesiku and D.E. McMahon have nothing to disclose.

REFERENCES

1. Karimkhani C, Dellavalle RP, Coffeng LE, et al. Global skin disease morbidity and mortality: an update from the Global Burden of Disease Study 2013. JAMA Dermatol 2017;153(5):406–12.
2. Seth D, Cheldize K, Brown D, et al. Global burden of skin disease: inequities and innovations. Curr Dermatol Rep 2017;6(3):204–10.
3. Lotti T, Handog EB, Hercogová J, et al. International dermatology: the many faces and challenges of the specialty in the global village. Dermatol Clin 2008; 26(2):183–90, v.
4. Ryan TJ. One of the greatest of health needs without effective advocacy and shamefully neglected! Br J Dermatol 2008;158(2):205–7.
5. McMichael J, Norton SA, Stoff BK. Interested in global health? Here is where to start: a checklist for United States dermatology residents. Int J Dermatol 2018;57(3):e23–6.
6. Freeman EE. A seat at the big table: expanding the role of dermatology at the World Health Organization and beyond. J Invest Dermatol 2014;134(11): 2663–5.
7. Drain PK, Primack A, Hunt DD, et al. Global health in medical education: a call for more training and opportunities. Acad Med 2007;82(3).
8. Hay RJ. Global dermatology: more than the sum of its parts. Br J Dermatol 2014;171(5):923–5.
9. Introcaso CE, Kovarik CL. Dermatology in Botswana: The American Academy of Dermatology's Resident International Grant. Dermatol Clin 2011;29(1):63–7.
10. Dixon CA, Castillo J, Castillo H, et al. Global health opportunities within pediatric subspecialty fellowship training programs: surveying the virtual landscape. BMC Med Educ 2013;13:88.
11. Nelson BD, Kasper J, Hibberd PL, et al. Developing a career in global health: considerations for physicians-in-training and academic mentors. J Grad Med Educ 2012;4(3):301–6.
12. Lipoff JB, Jariwala N, Paz M, et al. Establishment of a dermatology global health outreach and residency partnership program in Guatemala. J Am Acad Dermatol 2017;76(5):993–4.e1.
13. Fuller LC, Hay RJ. Global health dermatology: building community, gaining momentum. Br J Dermatol 2019;180(6):1279–80.
14. Laker-Oketta MO, Wenger M, Semeere A, et al. Task shifting and skin punch for the histologic diagnosis of Kaposi's sarcoma in Sub-Saharan Africa: a public health solution to a public health problem. Oncology 2015;89(1):60–5.
15. Hay RC, Olivier C, Naldi L, et al. WHO approval of a new essential medicine for dermatology – oral ivermectin. 2019. Available at: https://ilds.org/news/approval-eml-ivermectin/. Accessed May 11, 2020.
16. WHO. Scabies and other ectoparasites. 2020. Available at: https://www.who.int/neglected_diseases/diseases/scabies-and-other-ectoparasites/en/. Accessed May 11, 2020.
17. WHO. Guidelines on the treatment of skin and oral HIV-associated conditions in children and adults. Geneva (Switzerland): WHO; 2014. 9789241548915.
18. WHO. Recognizing neglected tropical diseases through changes on the skin: a training guide for front-line health workers. Geneva (Switzerland): WHO; 2018.
19. WHO. Epidemiology and management of common skin diseases in children in developing countries. Geneva (Switzerland): WHO; 2005.
20. Coates SJ, McCalmont TH, Williams ML. Adapting to the effects of climate change in the practice of dermatology—a call to action. JAMA Dermatol 2019;155(4):415–6.
21. Fuller LC, Hay R, Morrone A, et al. Guidelines on the role of skin care in the management of mobile populations. Int J Dermatol 2013;52(2):200–8.
22. Hay RJ, Augustin M, Griffiths CEM, et al. the Board of the International League of Dermatological S, the Grand Challenges Consultation g. The global challenge for skin health. Br J Dermatol 2015; 172(6):1469–72.
23. Hay RJ. The role of international dermatology organizations. Clin Dermatol 2012;30(6):668–71.
24. Lonowski SL, Rodriguez O, Carlos CA, et al. Looking back on 10 years of the American Academy of Dermatology's Resident International Grant Experience in Botswana. J Am Acad Dermatol 2019. S0190-9622(19)33312-2. https://doi.org/10.1016/j.jaad.2019.12.035.
25. Evensen A, Duffy S, Dawe R, et al. Status of global health fellowship training in the United States and Canada. Can Med Educ J 2019;10(4):e80–95.
26. Drain PK, Holmes KK, Skeff KM, et al. Global health training and international clinical rotations during residency: current status, needs, and opportunities. Acad Med 2009;84(3):320–5.
27. Amir M, Sampson BP, Endly D, et al. Social networking sites: emerging and essential tools for

communication in dermatology. JAMA Dermatol 2014;150(1):56–60.

28. Lescano AG, Cohen CR, Raj T, et al. Strengthening mentoring in low- and middle-income countries to advance global health research: an overview. Am J Trop Med Hyg 2019;100(1_Suppl):3–8.

29. Bennett S, Paina L, Ssengooba F, et al. Mentorship in African health research training programs: an exploratory study of Fogarty International Center Programs in Kenya and Uganda. Educ Health (Abingdon) 2013;26(3):183–7.

30. John CC, Ayodo G, Musoke P. Successful global health research partnerships: what makes them work? Am J Trop Med Hyg 2016;94(1):5–7.

31. ISD. Corporate Partners. 2018. Available at: https://www.intsocderm.org/i4a/pages/index.cfm?pageID=3480&activateFull=true. Accessed May 12, 2020.

32. ILDS. About Us. 2020. Available at: https://ilds.org/about-us/. Accessed April 17, 2020.

33. RDTC. History. 2020. Available at: https://rdtc.go.tz/about-us/history/. Accessed April 17, 2020.

34. Comunitaria D. Our Goals. 2020. Available at: http://dermatologiacomunitaria.org.mx/goals.html. Accessed May 12, 2020.

35. Hay R, Andersson N, Estrada R. Mexico: community dermatology in Guerrero. Lancet 1991;337(8746):906–7.

36. International Society of Dermatology in the Tropics: Bylaws in English. 2020. Available at: https://www.tropendermatologie.de/EN/dokumente/bylaws-of-the-international.html. Accessed May 12, 2020.

37. IACS. About the International Alliance for the Control of Scabies. 2020. Available at: https://www.controlscabies.org/about-iacs. Accessed May 12, 2020.

38. Engelman D, Yoshizumi J, Hay RJ, et al. The 2020 International Alliance for the Control of Scabies Consensus Criteria for the Diagnosis of Scabies. Br J Dermatol 2020. https://doi.org/10.1111/bjd.18943.

Tools for Dermatology Care in Resource Limited Settings:

Novel Diagnostics for Kaposi Sarcoma and Other Skin Diseases in Resource-Limited Settings

Devon E. McMahon, BA[a], Linda Oyesiku, MPH[b,c],
Aggrey Semeere, MBChB, MMED, MAS[d], Dongkyun Kang, PhD[e],
Esther E. Freeman, MD, PhD[a,*]

KEYWORDS

- Point of care • Delayed diagnosis • Dermatology • Dermatopathology • Kaposi sarcoma
- Cutaneous leishmaniasis • Leprosy • Buruli ulcer • Yaws • Onchocerciasis

KEY POINTS

- Point-of-care diagnostics are uniquely suited to address diagnostic delays for many dermatologic conditions in resource limited settings.
- Novel devices have been developed to aid the diagnosis of Kaposi sarcoma, cutaneous leishmaniasis, leprosy, Buruli ulcer, yaws, onchocerciasis, and lymphatic filariasis.
- Although there are multiple prototypes of these devices for a variety of dermatologic conditions, there remain many barriers to implementation, including validation, cost, scale, and sustainability.

INTRODUCTION

In resource-limited settings, there are multiple factors that lead to diagnostic delays for dermatologic conditions **Table 1**. First, there are limited numbers of dermatologists in these settings, with estimates of 1 dermatologist per 1 million people in urban sub-Saharan Africa and even fewer in rural areas.[1] This lack of specialists leads to many dermatologic diagnoses being made by front-line providers who often lack dermatologic training.[2–4] Next, obtaining traditional dermatopathology and laboratory services is difficult owing to a lack of dermatologists, surgical equipment, pathologists trained in dermatopathology, histopathology, laboratories and supplies.[5,6] Additionally, patients must often travel substantial distances and pay considerable fees to obtain a diagnosis, leading to a large number of patients who are lost to follow-up after the initial visit.[7–9] These factors all lead to the delayed diagnosis of dermatologic diseases, some of which are more severe with poor treatment outcomes after such delays.[10–12]

Point-of-care (POC) devices have the potential to alleviate these issues by providing same-day diagnosis by a nonspecialized provider without the need for advanced pathology or laboratory equipment.[13] However, the design and implementation of novel POC technologies in resource-limited settings has many challenges. Devices must be low cost, not require highly specialized workers, be easy to transport, and not require highly equipped laboratories.[13,14] Additionally, in many settings devices must be able to work without electricity and be stored in a wide range of temperatures. There are further financial challenges to product development, given the

^a Department of Dermatology, Harvard Medical School, Massachusetts General Hospital, 50 Staniford Street, Boston, MA 02114, USA; ^b Department of Dermatology, Massachusetts General Hospital, 50 Staniford Street, Boston, MA 02114, USA; ^c University of Miami Miller School of Medicine, Miami, FL, USA; ^d Infectious Diseases Institute, Kampala, Uganda; ^e University of Arizona, Tucson, AZ, USA
* Corresponding author.
E-mail address: efreeman@mgh.harvard.edu

Dermatol Clin 39 (2021) 83–90
https://doi.org/10.1016/j.det.2020.08.008
0733-8635/21/© 2020 Elsevier Inc. All rights reserved.

derm.theclinics.com

Table 1
Novel devices for point-of-care diagnosis of dermatologic conditions designed for resource limited settings.

Device	Brief Description	Sensitivity[a]	Specificity[a]	Stage of Development
Kaposi sarcoma				
TINY	LAMP device to detect Kaposi sarcoma herpesvirus	93%	94%	Prototype; field testing
Portable Reflective Confocal Microscopy	Low-cost confocal microscope to noninvasively image dermis	—	—	Prototype; field testing
Cutaneous Leishmaniasis				
SpeedXtract/RPA	Uses RPA on a quick 2 mm punch biopsy extraction obtained via SpeedXtract	65.5%	100%	Prototype; field testing
Loopamp	Uses LAMP to detect a conserved gene across *Leishmania* species	91.4%	91.7%	Prototype; field testing
CL Detect Rapid Test	An immunochromatographic test to detect the peroxidoxin antigen of *Leishmania* on a test strip	35.8%	83.3%	Prototype; field testing
Mycobacterium Leprae				
Upconverting phosphor lateral flow assay	Uses upconverting phosphor lateral flow assays to detect leprosy biomarkers including anti–phenolic glycolipid-I antibodies, IFN-γ induced protein 10, and additional immune markers CCL4, IL-10, and CRP	75%–97%	—	Prototype; field testing
Buruli Ulcer				
LAMP assays	LAMP device for *M. ulcerans* skin biopsies	83.8% - 86.8%	100%	Prototype; field testing
M ulcerans RPA (Mu-RPA)	RPA device for *M. ulcerans* detection with fine needle aspirates or swabs	88%	100%	Prototype
Thin Layer Chromatography to Detect Mycolactone	Uses fluorescent thin layer chromatography to detect the *M. ulcerans* toxin mycolactone	73.2%	85.7%	Prototype
Yaws				
The Dual Path Platform	Detects antibodies to treponemal and nontreponemal antigens in settings without electricity or running water	88.4%	95.2%	Prototype; field testing
Onchocerciasis				
LoaScope	Smartphone video microscope to detect Loa loa microfilariae	—	99.7%	Field testing; production
Lymphatic Filariasis				
The Alere Filariasis Test Strip	Detects filarial antigens of *Wuchereria bancrofti*	94.9%	84.0%	Field testing; production

[a] Compared with current standard of care diagnostic device.

estimated cost of $2 million to $10 million for POC device development over a 5- to 10-year period.[14] Because the production of diagnostic tests is largely driven by the private sector in high-income countries, for diseases that are more common in low-resource settings, there are fewer funding sources.[14]

Since the turn of the millennium, several remarkable advances in POC diagnostics in many medical fields have been made. Overcoming these challenges with new technology seems to be the main approach. This effect has been referred to as the leapfrog effect, whereby certain technology advances can jump-start development by bypassing system impediments. An example of the leapfrog effect for POC diagnostics is a laboratory on a chip micro-fluid technologies using lateral flow enzyme immunoassays, which have allowed for the diagnosis of many diseases before a traditional laboratory has been established. Examples of their use include protein analysis (ie, anti–human immunodeficiency virus antibodies), nucleic acid analysis (ie, human immunodeficiency virus, hepatitis B, tuberculosis), cell counting (ie, complete blood count), and blood chemistries (ie, electrolytes, blood gas).[15–17] Although these microfluid technologies are inexpensive and easy to use, they are generally less sensitive than nucleic acid amplification assays (NAATs), such as polymerase chain reaction (PCR)[13] and hence could benefit from further optimization. More recently, isothermal NAAT techniques have been developed that can be performed at a single temperature and with minimal instrumentation.[13] An example of novel NAAT technologies are recombinase polymerase assay (RPA) and loop-mediated isothermal amplification (LAMP), which often approach the sensitivity of PCR testing but in a shorter time frame and with fewer laboratory requirements.[18] Because RPA and LAMP are performed at a single temperature, they can be executed using simple instruments and alternative heating sources to electricity.

POC diagnostic devices are not new concepts in dermatology. Diagnostic tools such as potassium hydroxide preparation for superficial mycoses and slit skin smear for leprosy have been available for many decades and continue to be quick and cost-effective diagnostic tools in both resource-rich and resource-limited settings.[19] In this article, we outline novel POC diagnostics for dermatologic conditions which primarily affect patients living in resource limited settings: Kaposi sarcoma, cutaneous leishmaniasis, leprosy, Buruli ulcer, yaws, onchocerciasis, and lymphatic filariasis (**Table 1**).

NOVEL DIAGNOSTICS
Kaposi Sarcoma

Kaposi sarcoma is an AIDS-defining malignancy that is one of the most prevalent cancers in Eastern and Southern Africa.[20] The majority of patients present with advanced disease, which necessitates chemotherapy and portends poor overall survival.[21] A study found that on average patients with Kaposi sarcoma visit 3 clinical providers before obtaining a histopathologic diagnosis.[22] Barriers to diagnosis are likely related to gaps in provider and patient knowledge of Kaposi sarcoma presentation, lack of access to histopathology, and patient's inability to pay for histopathology.[22] Additionally, in many locations Kaposi sarcoma continues to be diagnosed by clinical means alone, leading to patients inappropriately receiving treatment for Kaposi sarcoma.[5] A same-day POC test could potentially alleviate many of these issues, and furthermore provide a screening test for all patients with human immunodeficiency virus who present with new cutaneous lesions.[23] Prototypes of 2 such devices with the potential to reduce delays in Kaposi sarcoma diagnosis have recently been developed and are currently being tested.

Tiny isothermal nucleic acid quantification system

Tiny isothermal nucleic acid quantification system (TINY) is a portable device that uses LAMP to quantitatively detect the amount of Kaposi sarcoma-causing virus, Kaposi sarcoma herpesvirus, which is also known as human herpesvirus 8, in skin or the mucosal tissue (**Fig. 1**).[24] The device is inexpensive ($250 USD) and can be used with multiple energy sources, including sunlight, electricity, and flame. When TINY was used in optimal settings at US laboratories and compared with US-based dermatopathology as a gold standard, the device had a sensitivity of 93% and a specificity of 94%.[25] Presently TINY is being validated in real-world settings in sub-Saharan Africa. A drawback of TINY is that it still requires a skin biopsy, which continues to be inaccessible and expensive in many countries.[6]

Portable reflective confocal microscopy

A POC device for Kaposi sarcoma that could potentially bypass the need for skin biopsy all-together is reflectance confocal microscopy. Reflectance confocal microscopy technology is already used for skin cancers in resource-rich settings to noninvasively visualize the epidermis and papillary dermis.[26] Although the diagnosis of Kaposi sarcoma with reflectance confocal microscopy is a possibility, the prohibitively high cost

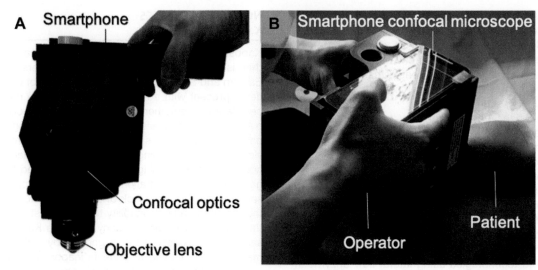

Fig. 1. (*A*) Portable confocal microscope for POC Kaposi sarcoma diagnosis using a smartphone. (*B*) Field testing of smartphone confocal microscope on a patient.

of RCM (approximately $100,000 USD) makes it untenable for use in low-resource environments.[27,28] A portable smartphone confocal microscope has been engineered to capture images from a microscope on a smartphone at a lower cost of $4200 USD.[29] Preliminary testing of this device in Uganda showed that the device was efficient and easy to use by midlevel providers.[26] However, whether or not the device can be used to distinguish Kaposi sarcoma from mimickers remains to be demonstrated; image analysis is ongoing.[26] High-quality image capture with a smartphone can plug into the growing potential for artificial intelligence to provide a diagnosis for various conditions.

Cutaneous Leishmaniasis

Leishmaniasis is a neglected tropical disease caused by *Leishmania donovani*, a protozoan parasite transmitted to humans by an infected sand fly. Leishmaniasis causes a range of dermatologic diseases, including chronic nonhealing ulcers. Diagnosis of cutaneous leishmaniasis requires laboratory confirmation, which usually entails high-cost PCR in resource-rich settings or the inexpensive Giemsa-stained slit skin smear, which has a low sensitivity.[30] Early treatment is critical to prevent enlargement of scars and to decrease the risk of developing visceral leishmaniasis.

SpeedXtract/recombinase polymerase assay
A POC mobile laboratory was developed to combine a quick DNA extraction (SpeedXtract) with a RPA detection method, with promising results for visceral leishminasis.[31] The same

procedure was then tested for cutaneous leishmaniasis in Sri Lanka, which used a 2 mm punch biopsy and toothpick to perform the SpeedXtract DNA extraction process. When tested against conventional PCR techniques, SpeedXtract/RPA had a sensitivity of 65.5%, compared with 32.2% for Giemsa-stained slit skin smear, which is often used in resource-limited settings.[30] Additionally, whereas conventional PCR techniques took 8 hours to perform, SpeedXtract/RPA was performed in 35 minutes. There were challenges with the method of sample transportation, and additional studies are required to validate transportation and storage protocols.

Loopamp
Loopamp is a nucleic acid amplification test that uses LAMP to detect a conserved 18S rRNA gene of *Leishmania* species and a specific sequence in *L donovani*. Similar to the TINY device for Kaposi sarcoma, Loopamp requires DNA extraction via skin biopsy before the test can be performed. In one study, as compared with PCR, Loopamp had a sensitivity of 91.4% and specificity of 91.7%.[32] Loopmap has been tested in Suriname,[32] Columbia,[33] and Afghanistan[34] with comparable results even across variations in old world and new world *Leishmania* species.

CL Detect Rapid Test
The CL Detect Rapid Test is an immunochromatographic test that detects the peroxidoxin antigen of *Leishmania* species using a test strip. This POC device initially held promise as a way to rapidly obtain a tissue sample from a small dental broach and obtain results in less than 1 hour with

interpretation in the same manner as malaria rapid detection tests. However, when compared with PCR, this test only had a sensitivity of 35.8% and specificity of 83.3%.[32]

Mycobacterium leprae

Leprosy remains endemic in many low- and middle-income countries, causing significant morbidity from nerve and skin damage. Patients infected with Mycobacterium leprae, the causative agent of leprosy, can develop a range of immune responses ranging from a strong Th1 tuberculoid response to a strong Th2 lepromatous response.[35] Most patients are diagnosed on clinical grounds or with slit-skin smear when available, but these tests often miss patients with paucibacillary disease.

Upconverting phosphor lateral flow assay for leprosy

Novel PCR methods have been developed for the diagnosis of M leprae either from a skin biopsy or slit skin smear; however, there continue to be concerns about their sensitivity, specificity, and cost.[36] These diagnostic tests either rely on high IgM against phenolic glycolipid I, which do not identify paucibacillary cases, or rely on enzyme-linked immunosorbent assay techniques to determine IFN-γ production, which require advanced laboratory facilities.[35] Using low-tech, low-cost upconverting phosphor lateral flow assays, researchers have developed a POC device to detect both anti–phenolic glycolipid-I antibodies as markers of humoral immunity, as well as IFN-γ–induced protein 10, and additional immune markers CCL4, IL-10, and CRP as markers of cellular immunity.[35] This method has been validated as improving the detection of both multibacillary and particularly paucibacillary leprosy across the globe including in Bangladesh, China, Brazil, and Ethiopia.[35,37] Testing so far has shown a sensitivity of 75% to 97% for patients with lepromatous leprosy and 71% to 80% for tuberculoid leprosy.[37] This test can additionally be performed with finger stick blood tests, allowing for increased ease of testing.[38]

Buruli Ulcer

Buruli ulcer is a neglected tropical disease caused by Mycobacterium ulcerans that causes painful and disfiguring ulcerative lesions. Although PCR to detect IS2404 sequence of M ulcerans is the most sensitive method to diagnose Buruli ulcer, PCR is costly and often not available in many laboratories in resource-limited settings. The following POC tests have been developed to address this gap.

Loop-mediated isothermal amplification assays for M ulcerans

Multiple groups have developed LAMP assay for M ulcerans, which perform similarly to standard PCR in a variety of climates. For example, a LAMP study on samples from Togo and Ghana showed a sensitivity of 86.8% and 83.8% respectively, as well as a specificity of 100% for 2 novel LAMP devices compared with PCR, at the lower cost of USD $1 to $2 per LAMP reaction.[39]

M ulcerans recombinase polymerase amplification

A POC test was developed using RPA of multiple strains of M ulcerans to rapidly diagnose Buruli ulcer using fine needle aspirates or swabs.[40] When compared with PCR, sensitivity was 88% and specificity was 100%.[40] So far this device has only been tested in ideal laboratory settings, so its efficacy in real-world settings remains to be seen.

Thin layer chromatography to detect mycolactone

Finally, an alternative non-NAAT based POC test using fluorescent thin layer chromatography has been developed to detect the M ulcerans toxin mycolactone. Compared with conventional PCR, thin layer chromatography had a sensitivity of 73.2% and specificity of 85.7%.[41] Samples were easily collected using fine needle aspiration or a tissue swab. This test has only been validated in optimal laboratory conditions, thus further testing in resource limited settings is needed.[41]

Yaws

Yaws is a neglected tropical disease caused by Treponema pallidum pertenue, and is a close relative of syphilis. Untreated, yaws can cause disseminated cutaneous lesions and destruction of bones, leading to significant morbidity. Owing to their similarity, yaws and syphilis can be tested using the same treponemal antigen and nontreponemal antigens tests.[42] Nontreponemal testing for yaws and syphilis such as rapid plasma regain is frequently unavailable in yaws-endemic areas and requires laboratory infrastructure.[43]

The dual path platform

A novel POC immunoassay called the dual path platform assay is able to detect antibodies to both treponemal and nontreponemal antigens in settings without electricity, running water, or laboratory equipment.[43] When compared with standard rapid plasma regain and Treponema pallidum haemagglutination assays, the dual path platform T1 (treponemal) assay had a sensitivity of 88.4% and specificity of 95.2%, whereas the dual path platform T2 (nontreponemal) assay had a sensitivity of 87.9% and specificity of 92.5% when tested on children in Papua New Guinea.[42]

Onchocerciasis and Lymphatic Filariasis

Onchocerciasis is a neglected tropical disease that causes rashes, pruritus, visual impairment, and blindness. Lymphatic filariasis is a common cause of elephantiasis, which causes significant disability and stigma in many low resource settings, of which around 90% of cases are caused by the parasite *Wuchereria bancrofti*.[44] Both onchocerciasis and *W bancrofti* lymphatic filariasis are common in Central Africa and treated with ivermectin. In Central Africa, mass drug administration of ivermectin is used to treat and eliminate *Loa loa*, causing onchocerciasis and *Onchocerca volvulus* causing lymphatic filariasis. However, around 5% of patients have high *L loa* microfilarial densities that, when treated with ivermectin, can cause serious adverse neurologic events.[45]

LoaScope

To prevent the adverse events of high *L loa* microfilarial densities, a POC smartphone-based video-microscope called the LoaScope was developed to screen the peripheral blood of patients for high densities of *L loa* microfilariae.[46] When the LoaScope was tested in Cameroon as part of a test-and-not-treat program for mass ivermectin administration, patients had fewer ivermectin-associated adverse events.[45] Additionally, the LoaScope had a specificity of 99.7% when compared with traditional thick blood smear microscopy.[45]

The Alere Filariasis test strip

To assess the burden of filariasis and success of mass drug administration of ivermectin, the Alere Filariasis Test Strip has been developed. It is a qualitative POC test that can detect the circulating filarial antigens of *W bancrofti* with finger-prick blood samples.[47] This method allows for a same-day low-cost diagnostic test, which avoids the laboratory requirements and high costs of traditional enzyme-linked immunosorbent assay testing.

SUMMARY

By providing more rapid and accurate diagnoses, investments in POC devices have the potential to improve time to diagnosis, treatment initiation, and epidemiologic surveillance of dermatologic diseases. However, there are a large number of common dermatologic disorders in resource limited settings that do not yet have procedures for POC diagnosis. Furthermore, there are multiple steps from validation of a POC prototype, to real-world POC validation, and the actual purchase, installation, and maintenance of these devices in clinics and hospitals in resource-limited settings. These next steps require evaluation through implementation science, and partnering with national ministries of health and existing donor structures to improve their availability. Of note, none of the diagnostic tests described in this article have been placed on the World Health Organization Model List of Essential In Vitro Diagnostics, which to date does not have any devices specifically for dermatologic conditions.[48] Additional diagnostic aids, including teledermatology and training mid-level providers in dermatologic diagnosis, will likely be necessary to improve dermatologic diagnosis.[6,49] Looking to the future, artificial intelligence may be a technologic advance that could potentially provide a POC screening tool or even diagnosis for all dermatologic conditions discussed in this article, and many more.[50]

CLINICS CARE POINTS

- Many dermatologic conditions are well suited to be diagnosed with point-of-care devices. Novel devices may be particularly important in resource limited settings especially those where specialists and traditional dermatopathology are unavailable.

DISCLOSURE

Dr. Freeman's effort was supported by the National Institutes of Health (K23 AI136579). E.E. Freeman and A. Semeere are investigators on UH3CA202723 and R21TW010221 to study the implementation of the TINY and portable confocal microscopy technologies discussed in this article. D. Kang is an investigator of R21TW010221 to study the portable confocal microscope and is an inventor on a US patent (Massachusetts General Hospital, assignee) for the microscope. D.E. McMahon and L. Oyesiku have no conflicts of interest to disclose.

REFERENCES

1. Desai B, McKoy K, Kovarik C. Overview of international teledermatology. Pan Afr Med J 2010;6:3.
2. Hu J, McKoy K, Papier A, et al. Dermatology and HIV/AIDS in Africa. J Glob Infect Dis 2011;3(3):275–80.
3. George AO, Daramola OO. Dermatology in Nigeria: evolution, establishment and current status. Int J Dermatol 2004;43(3):223–8.

4. Brown DN, Langan SM, Freeman EE. Task shifting in dermatology: a call to action. JAMA Dermatol 2017; 153(11):1179–80.

5. Amerson E, Woodruff CM, Forrestel A, et al. Accuracy of clinical suspicion and pathologic diagnosis of Kaposi sarcoma in East Africa. J Acquir Immune Defic Syndr 2016;71(3):295–301.

6. Laker-Oketta MO, Wenger M, Semeere A, et al. Task shifting and skin punch for the histologic diagnosis of Kaposi's sarcoma in Sub-Saharan Africa: a public health solution to a public health problem. Oncology 2015;89(1):60–5.

7. Semeere A, Ayanga R, Freeman E, et al. What happens after the biopsy? Pace and determinants of the communication of pathology results to patients with suspected Kaposi's sarcoma in Uganda. 17th international conference on malignancies in HIV/AIDS; October 21-22, 2019; Bethesda (MD).

8. Williams VL, Narasimhamurthy M, Rodriguez O, et al. Dermatology-driven quality improvement interventions to decrease diagnostic delays for Kaposi sarcoma in Botswana. J Glob Oncol 2019;5:1–7.

9. Freeman E, Semeere A, Wenger M, et al. Pitfalls of practicing cancer epidemiology in resource-limited settings: the case of survival and loss to follow-up after a diagnosis of Kaposi's sarcoma in five countries across sub-Saharan Africa. BMC cancer 2016;16:65.

10. Cesarman E, Damania B, Krown SE, et al. Kaposi sarcoma. Nat Rev Dis Primers 2019;5(1):9.

11. Barogui YT, Sopoh GE, Johnson RC, et al. Contribution of the community health volunteers in the control of Buruli ulcer in Benin. PLoS Negl Trop Dis 2014; 8(10):e3200.

12. Chu T, Liu D, Huai P, et al. Comprehensive measures succeeded in improving early detection of leprosy cases in post-elimination era: experience from Shandong province, China. PLoS Negl Trop Dis 2020; 14(2):e0007891.

13. Hansen GT. Point-of-care testing in microbiology: a mechanism for improving patient outcomes. Clin Chem 2019;66(1):124–37.

14. Peeling RW, Mabey D. Point-of-care tests for diagnosing infections in the developing world. Clin Microbiol Infect 2010;16(8):1062–9.

15. Nasseri B, Soleimani N, Rabiee N, et al. Point-of-care microfluidic devices for pathogen detection. Biosens Bioelectron 2018;117:112–28.

16. Chin CD, Linder V, Sia SK. Lab-on-a-chip devices for global health: past studies and future opportunities. Lab Chip 2007;7(1):41–57.

17. Diaconu K, Chen YF, Cummins C, et al. Methods for medical device and equipment procurement and prioritization within low- and middle-income countries: findings of a systematic literature review. Global Health 2017;13(1):59.

18. LaBarre P, Hawkins KR, Gerlach J, et al. A simple, inexpensive device for nucleic acid amplification without electricity-toward instrument-free molecular diagnostics in low-resource settings. PLoS One 2011;6(5):e19738.

19. Wanat KA, Dominguez AR, Carter Z, et al. Bedside diagnostics in dermatology: viral, bacterial, and fungal infections. J Am Acad Dermatol 2017;77(2): 197–218.

20. Bray F, Ferlay J, Soerjomataram I, et al. Global cancer statistics 2018: GLOBOCAN estimates of incidence and mortality worldwide for 36 cancers in 185 countries. CA Cancer J Clin 2018;68(6): 394–424.

21. Okuku F, Krantz EM, Kafeero J, et al. Evaluation of a predictive staging model for HIV-associated Kaposi sarcoma in Uganda. J Acquir Immune Defic Syndr 2017;74(5):548–54.

22. Laker-Oketta M, Busakhala N, Byakwaga H, et al. Why are they diagnosed so late? Understanding the circumstances preceding diagnosis among patients with Kaposi's sarcoma identified by rapid case ascertainment in East Africa. 17th international conference on malignancies in HIV/AIDS; October 21-22, 2019; Bethesda (MD).

23. McMahon DE, Maurer T, Freeman EE. 25 years of Kaposi sarcoma herpesvirus: discoveries, disparities, and diagnostics. JCO Glob Oncol 2020;6: 505–7.

24. Snodgrass R, Gardner A, Semeere A, et al. A portable device for nucleic acid quantification powered by sunlight, a flame or electricity. Nat Biomed Eng 2018;2(9):657–65.

25. Martin J, Semeere A, Snodgrass R, et al. Employing the virus alone to diagnose the cancer: quantification of lesional KSHV DNA for the diagnosis of Kaposi's sarcoma in Africa. 17th international conference on malignancies in HIV/AIDS; October 21-22, 2019; Bethesda (MD).

26. Freeman EE, Semeere A, Laker-Oketta M, et al. Feasibility and implementation of portable confocal microscopy for point-of-care diagnosis of cutaneous lesions in a low-resource setting. J Am Acad Dermatol 2020. https://doi.org/10.1016/j.jaad.2020.04.147.

27. Grazziotin TC, Cota C, Buffon RB, et al. Preliminary evaluation of in vivo reflectance confocal microscopy features of Kaposi's sarcoma. Dermatology 2010;220(4):346–54.

28. Pellacani G, Witkowski A, Cesinaro AM, et al. Cost-benefit of reflectance confocal microscopy in the diagnostic performance of melanoma. J Eur Acad Dermatol Venereol 2016;30(3):413–9.

29. Freeman EE, Semeere A, Osman H, et al. Smartphone confocal microscopy for imaging cellular structures in human skin in vivo. Biomed Opt Express 2018;9(4):1906–15.

30. Gunaratna G, Manamperi A, Bohlken-Fascher S, et al. Evaluation of rapid extraction and isothermal amplification techniques for the detection of

Leishmania donovani DNA from skin lesions of suspected cases at the point of need in Sri Lanka. Parasit Vectors 2018;11(1):665.

31. Mondal D, Ghosh P, Khan MA, et al. Mobile suitcase laboratory for rapid detection of Leishmania donovani using recombinase polymerase amplification assay. Parasit Vectors 2016;9(1):281.

32. Schallig H, Hu RVP, Kent AD, et al. Evaluation of point of care tests for the diagnosis of cutaneous leishmaniasis in Suriname. BMC Infect Dis 2019; 19(1):25.

33. Adams ER, Schoone G, Versteeg I, et al. Development and evaluation of a novel loop-mediated isothermal amplification assay for diagnosis of cutaneous and visceral leishmaniasis. J Clin Microbiol 2018;56(7). e00386-18.

34. Vink MMT, Nahzat SM, Rahimi H, et al. Evaluation of point-of-care tests for cutaneous leishmaniasis diagnosis in Kabul, Afghanistan. EBioMedicine 2018;37: 453–60.

35. Bobosha K, Tjon Kon Fat EM, van den Eeden SJ, et al. Field-evaluation of a new lateral flow assay for detection of cellular and humoral immunity against Mycobacterium leprae. PLoS Negl Trop Dis 2014;8(5):e2845.

36. Tatipally S, Srikantam A, Kasetty S. Polymerase chain reaction (PCR) as a potential point of care laboratory test for leprosy diagnosis-a systematic review. Trop Med Infect Dis 2018;3(4):107.

37. van Hooij A, Tjon Kon Fat EM, Batista da Silva M, et al. Evaluation of immunodiagnostic tests for leprosy in Brazil, China and Ethiopia. Sci Rep 2018;8(1):17920.

38. Corstjens P, van Hooij A, Tjon Kon Fat EM, et al. Fingerstick test quantifying humoral and cellular biomarkers indicative for M. leprae infection. Clin Biochem 2019;66:76–82.

39. Beissner M, Phillips RO, Battke F, et al. Loop-mediated isothermal amplification for laboratory confirmation of buruli ulcer disease-towards a point-of-care test. PLoS Negl Trop Dis 2015;9(11):e0004219.

40. Frimpong M, Ahor HS, Wahed AAE, et al. Rapid detection of mycobacterium ulcerans with isothermal recombinase polymerase amplification assay. PLoS Negl Trop Dis 2019;13(2):e0007155.

41. Wadagni A, Frimpong M, Phanzu DM, et al. Simple, rapid mycobacterium ulcerans disease diagnosis from clinical samples by fluorescence of mycolactone on thin layer chromatography. PLoS Negl Trop Dis 2015;9(11):e0004247.

42. Ayove T, Houniei W, Wangnapi R, et al. Sensitivity and specificity of a rapid point-of-care test for active yaws: a comparative study. Lancet Glob Health 2014;2(7):e415–21.

43. Yin YP, Chen XS, Wei WH, et al. A dual point-of-care test shows good performance in simultaneously detecting nontreponemal and treponemal antibodies in patients with syphilis: a multisite evaluation study in China. Clin Infect Dis 2013;56(5):659–65.

44. Rebollo MP, Bockarie MJ. Shrinking the lymphatic filariasis map: update on diagnostic tools for mapping and transmission monitoring. Parasitology 2014;141(14):1912–7.

45. Kamgno J, Pion SD, Chesnais CB, et al. A test-and-not-treat strategy for onchocerciasis in loa loa-endemic areas. N Engl J Med 2017;377(21): 2044–52.

46. D'Ambrosio MV, Bakalar M, Bennuru S, et al. Point-of-care quantification of blood-borne filarial parasites with a mobile phone microscope. Sci Transl Med 2015;7(286):286re284.

47. Chesnais CB, Vlaminck J, Kunyu-Shako B, et al. Measurement of circulating filarial antigen levels in human blood with a point-of-care test strip and a portable spectrodensitometer. Am J Trop Med Hyg 2016;94(6):1324–9.

48. Second WHO Model list of essential in Vitro diagnostics. Available at: https://www.who.int/medical_devices/publications/Standalone_document_v8.pdf?ua=1. Accessed March 8, 2020.

49. Lipoff JB, Cobos G, Kaddu S, et al. The Africa teledermatology project: a retrospective case review of 1229 consultations from sub-Saharan Africa. J Am Acad Dermatol 2015;72(6):1084–5.

50. Esteva A, Kuprel B, Novoa RA, et al. Dermatologist-level classification of skin cancer with deep neural networks. Nature 2017;542(7639):115–8.

Implementing a Locally Made Low-Cost Intervention for Wound and Lymphedema Care in Western Kenya

Aileen Y. Chang, MD[a,b,*], Margaret Mungai, BSN[c], Sarah J. Coates, MD[a,d], Tiffany Chao, BS[e], Haji Philip Odhiambo[a], Phelix M. Were, BS[a], Sara L. Fletcher, PharmD, MPH[f], Toby Maurer, MD[a,g], Rakhi Karwa, PharmD[a,h], Sonak D. Pastakia, PharmD, MPH, PhD[a,h]

KEYWORDS

- Africa • Kenya • Wound care • Lymphedema • Bullous drug reaction • Resource-limited setting
- Low- and middle-income countries • Revolving fund pharmacy

KEY POINTS

- Major barriers to provision of wound and lymphedema care in Western Kenya include availability, affordability, and accessibility of bandages.
- At Academic Model Providing Access to Healthcare (AMPATH) in Western Kenya, dermatologists and pharmacists collaborated to develop a 2-component compression bandage modeled after the Unna boot using locally available materials that cost 2 to 3 USD and is distributed through a revolving fund pharmacy network.
- Venous leg ulcers, traumatic leg ulcers, and leg lymphedema from Kaposi sarcoma are treated with the compression bandages; neuropathic ulcers and bullous drug eruptions are also treated with the bandages, without compression.
- In partnership with nursing, use of these bandages at the national referral hospital and a few county facilities has increased, but expanded utilization to a much larger catchment area is needed.

INTRODUCTION

In Western Kenya, the burden of chronic wounds and lymphedema has a significant impact on functionality and quality of life, driven by physical discomfort, impaired mobility, and foul odor. The epidemiology of chronic leg ulcers in sub-Saharan Africa is limited. In other regions of the world, chronic leg ulcers are common, with 60% of leg ulcers present for more than 6 months, and one-third persisting for more than 1 year.[1] In

[a] Academic Model Providing Access to Healthcare (AMPATH), Eldoret, Kenya; [b] Department of Dermatology, University of California, School of Medicine, P.O. Box 4606 Eldoret, Kenya 30100; [c] Clinical Services, Moi Teaching & Referral Hospital, PO Box 3, Code 30100, Eldoret, Kenya; [d] Department of Dermatology, University of California, San Francisco School of Medicine, 1701 Divisadero Street, Suite 4-20, San Francisco, CA 94143-0316, USA; [e] University of California, Irvine School of Medicine, 1001 Health Sciences Road, Irvine, CA 92617, USA; [f] Drug Use Research and Management, Oregon State University College of Pharmacy, 2730 SW Moody Avenue, CL5CP, Portland, OR 97201, USA; [g] Indiana University School of Medicine, 545 Barnhill Drive, Emerson Hall 139, Indianapolis, IN 46202, USA; [h] Purdue University College of Pharmacy, Fifth Third Bank Building, 640 Eskenazi Avenue, Indianapolis, IN 46202-2879, USA
* Corresponding author. 1001 Potrero, Building 90, Ward 92, San Francisco, CA 94110.
E-mail address: aileen.chang@ucsf.edu

Dermatol Clin 39 (2021) 91–100
https://doi.org/10.1016/j.det.2020.08.009
0733-8635/21/© 2020 Elsevier Inc. All rights reserved.

derm.theclinics.com

addition to venous stasis ulcers and diabetic ulcers, in sub-Saharan Africa, there is a high burden of traumatic soft tissue injuries[2–5] and thus traumatic wounds contribute to the burden of chronic leg ulcers. With lymphedema, there is also progressive functional impairment leading to disfiguring changes, skin hardening from fibrosis, and recurrent skin infections. These are associated with mental health illness,[6–8] social stigma,[9,10] poor quality of life,[11,12] and economic burden.[13–17]

Major barriers to provision of wound and lymphedema care in Western Kenya, as in other regions of sub-Saharan Africa, include availability, affordability, and accessibility. Compression therapy is the well-established standard of care for chronic leg ulcers from venous disease and lymphedema.[18,19] Prepackaged compression bandages used for wound and lymphedema management in resource-replete settings are cost-prohibitive, 7 to 20 USD exclusive of import taxes, and often not available. At Academic Model Providing Access to Healthcare (AMPATH) health centers in Western Kenya, 2 medical assistants, a dermatologist, and a primary care physician from Laguna Honda Hospital and Rehabilitation Center in San Francisco trained clinicians and nurses to apply donated, prepackaged compression bandages. After anecdotal observations that the donated 2-component compression bandages were effective in managing venous leg ulcers and lymphedema, AMPATH Dermatology and AMPATH Pharmacy collaborated to develop a sustainable local alternative.[20] AMPATH is a partnership between Moi Teaching & Referral Hospital (MTRH), Moi University College of Health Sciences, and a consortium of North American academic medical centers. AMPATH, a President's Emergency Plan for AIDS Relief-United States Agency for International Development (PEPFAR-USAID)-supported implementing partner, collaborates with the Ministry of Health (MOH) to serve a catchment area of more than 8 million people and has supported human immunodeficiency virus (HIV) care delivery for more than 165,000 patients at more than 500 sites across Western Kenya. Using the infrastructure and health care delivery model created through HIV care, AMPATH has been providing care for other chronic diseases, including diabetes, cancer, and dermatologic conditions.

Since 2017, locally available materials have been used to create an inexpensive, 2-component compression bandage in Kenya for 2 to 3 USD each,[20] modeled after the Unna boot. The first component is an inner paste bandage layer consisting of gauze impregnated with zinc oxide paste. The second component is an elastic crepe bandage, which can be applied with or without compression (**Fig. 1**). Trained pharmacists and pharmacy technicians assemble the 2-component compression bandages at MTRH, a public national referral hospital. Assembly time is 15 minutes per bandage. Bandage assembly is centralized to maintain quality assurance and preparation in a clean area to minimize the risk of contamination. These compression bandages are available for purchase at MTRH and also delivered to county and subcounty health facilities through the AMPATH revolving fund pharmacy network that supports the MOH pharmacies throughout Western Kenya. The revolving fund pharmacy model enables stable provision of medications and medical supplies by using revenue generated from sales to restock, thereby helping to ensure a reliable supply in the face of stock-outs at government facilities.[21]

Availability of affordable bandages has resulted in more patients seeking wound and lymphedema care at the MTRH Wound Clinic and several AMPATH-supported county and subcounty facilities. Since June 2018, 1200 compression bandages have been sold through the AMPATH revolving fund pharmacies at 3 sites across Western Kenya. An estimated 250 patients have been treated with these bandages. This expansion of wound and lymphedema care has led to training sessions on wound and lymphedema assessment and provision of adjuvant therapies, such as metronidazole gel, to address wound odor.[22,23] Moreover, providers have found additional uses for the bandages for conditions that require a protective bandage without compression, such as neuropathic ulcers and skin erosions caused by bullous drug eruptions. Before the development of these bandages, providers had extremely limited bandage options for protecting compromised skin.

Herein, we present a series of cases, including traumatic ulcer, venous stasis ulcer, lymphedema from Kaposi sarcoma, neuropathic ulcer, and bullous drug eruption, that have benefited from management with the aforementioned low-cost locally made bandages. We also reflect on key elements that have enabled successful

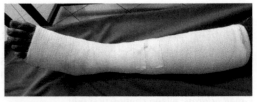

Fig. 1. Leg wrapped with locally made low-cost 2-component compression bandage.

implementation of this intervention and opportunities for scaling up this intervention across Western Kenya.

VENOUS STASIS ULCER

A 65-year-old woman presented with a history varicose veins and 5-year history of recurrent venous leg ulcers on the left medial and lateral leg (**Fig. 2**A, B). The wound was cleaned with normal saline and then mechanically debrided with a surgical blade and dissecting forceps. With the ankle joint positioned at 90°, a 2-component compression bandage was applied to the lower limb, starting from the mid-dorsum foot and ending just below the knee. Wound cleaning and compression bandage application occurred in clinic once to twice weekly. After several sessions, the patient's daughter, who is a nurse, was taught the compression bandage application technique to enable home-based care and reduce frequency of clinic visits. The patient was advised to return every 2 weeks for assessment or earlier for nonimprovement of wounds. On day 44, both medial and lateral wounds were completely healed (**Fig. 2**C, D). On discharge from the wound clinic,

the patient was advised to wear compression stockings.

TRAUMATIC ULCER

A 54-year-old woman presented with a 2-week history of a traumatic wound from a motorbike accident (**Fig. 3**A). Wet gauze bandages had been applied regularly at an outside hospital, but the patient had not observed any improvement. Following wound cleaning with normal saline, mechanical debridement using a surgical blade and dissecting forceps was performed, and a 2-component compression bandage was applied in clinic every 1 to 2 weeks. Four months later, the wound was completely healed (**Fig. 3**B). The patient reported having less pain and easier mobility.

LYMPHEDEMA FROM KAPOSI SARCOMA

A 44-year-old man presented with numerous skin nodules and large red tumors on a swollen right leg and foot (Campisi stage 3 lymphedema[24]). He complained of severe pain and odorous fluid draining from the tumors that impacted his activities of daily living and participation in social

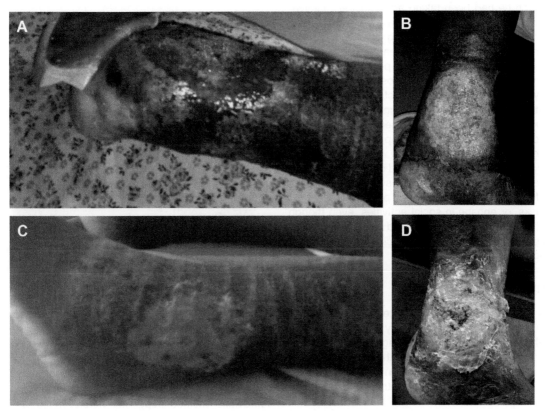

Fig. 2. Venous leg ulcer on the lateral left leg (*A*) and medial left leg (*B*) at initial presentation. After 44 days of compression therapy, healed ulcers on the lateral left leg (*C*) and medial left leg (*D*).

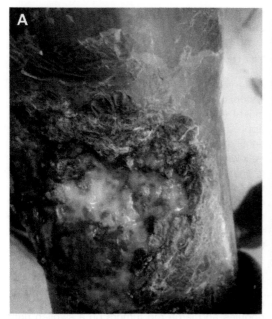
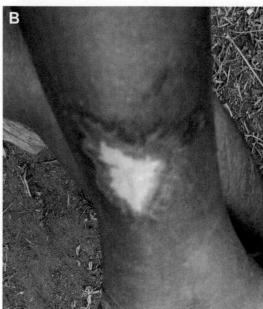

Fig. 3. Traumatic leg ulcer at initial presentation before debridement (*A*) and 4 months later when healed, leaving scar and dyspigmentation (*B*).

activities. Past medical history was notable for HIV (CD4 count and viral load were unknown), for which he had been taking antiretrovirals (lamivudine/tenofovir disoproxil fumarate/efavirenz) and cotrimoxazole for 2 years. Leg swelling had been present for approximately 2 years and skin lesions had developed 4 months prior. Skin biopsy confirmed a diagnosis of Kaposi sarcoma. After 8 cycles of bleomycin and vincristine chemotherapy, the tumors had improved significantly but lower extremity edema was still present. A 2-component compression bandage was applied in clinic and changed weekly. Following 10 weeks of compression therapy without continued chemotherapy, the patient noted that his leg swelling no longer affected his ability to walk, perform household tasks, or engage in social activities, even though photographs taken before and after the intervention do not reveal an appreciable difference in appearance (**Fig. 4**A–C).

NEUROPATHIC ULCER

A 75-year-old woman presented with an ulcer on the right heel of approximately 5 years' duration. She reported that 5 years ago she was diagnosed with malaria and treated with intramuscular quinine administered in the right gluteal muscle. A few days after treatment, the injection site was swollen and the right limb was numb. Intramuscular quinine is typically administered in the anterior thigh to avoid injury to the sciatic

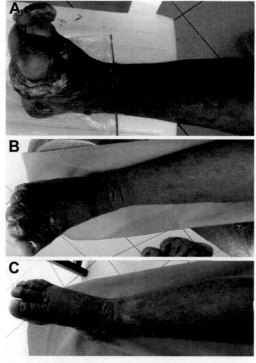

Fig. 4. Kaposi sarcoma lymphedema and tumors at initial presentation (*A*), after 8 cycles of bleomycin-vincristine chemotherapy, and before compression therapy (*B*), and after 10 weeks of compression therapy (*C*).

nerve, which can cause neuropathy. Soon thereafter, she observed an ulcer on the right heel. She denied a history of diabetes. The wound had been cared for with regular cleaning and dry gauze dressings every 2 to 3 days. This was intermittently accompanied by use of topical antibiotics and systemic antibiotics (exact medications unknown). On presentation to our clinic, the injection site swelling and numbness had subsided. Based on the history, appearance, and location of the ulcer, a diagnosis of neuropathic ulcer was made. The ulcer was cleaned with normal saline and metronidazole gel was applied to the ulcer base. Two-component bandages were applied from the dorsum of the foot at the point of the metatarsophalangeal joint to just above the lateral malleolus in clinic weekly. Bandages were applied without compression, as plantar pressure is believed to play an etiologic role in the development of neuropathic ulcers. After 10 weeks, the ulcer was healed (**Fig. 5**A, B).

BULLOUS DRUG REACTION

A 50-year-old woman presented with multifocal purpuric ovoid patches and sheets of sloughing skin without mucosal involvement that began 3 days before admission "immediately" after taking 2 doses of trimethoprim-sulfamethoxazole (TMP-SMX) for common cold symptoms (**Fig. 6**A). The patient noted that she frequently took TMP-SMX for common cold symptoms. TMP-SMX is a prescription drug in Kenya, but some pharmacies will dispense it without a prescription. She had no prior history of skin rashes or drug allergies. A diagnosis of generalized bullous fixed drug eruption was favored, and atypical Stevens Johnson Syndrome–Toxic Epidermolysis Necrosis was considered. A skin biopsy was not performed because the results would not alter management in this setting and the cost of histopathology specimen processing is 15 USD, which would have imposed a significant financial burden on this patient. TMP-SMX, the culprit drug, was stopped, and supportive care commenced. In the absence of alternative skin-directed therapies, the inner layer of the bandages (the zinc oxide–impregnated gauze layer) was applied to the denuded skin without compression. After 10 days, the patient's skin had reepithelialized (**Fig. 6**B).

DISCUSSION

Since the development of locally made low-cost bandages in Western Kenya, patients suffering from a range of wound and lymphedema etiologies have been successfully managed with these bandages. Patients with venous leg ulcers, traumatic leg ulcers, and leg lymphedema from Kaposi sarcoma have received compression with these bandages through tighter application of the outer layer elastic crepe component. Patients with neuropathic ulcers and bullous drug eruptions have received application of these bandages without compression.

Improvement of venous leg ulcers and leg lymphedema with compression bandages is consistent with this intervention being the standard of

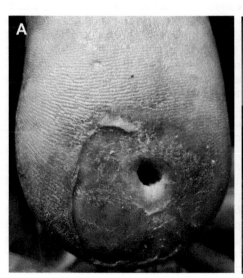
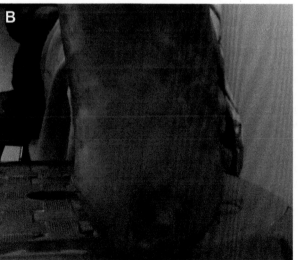

Fig. 5. Neuropathic ulcer on right heel at presentation (*A*) and 10 weeks after weekly ulcer cleaning, metronidazole gel, and application of 2-component bandages without compression (*B*). White substance is zinc oxide paste residue from the inner layer bandage.

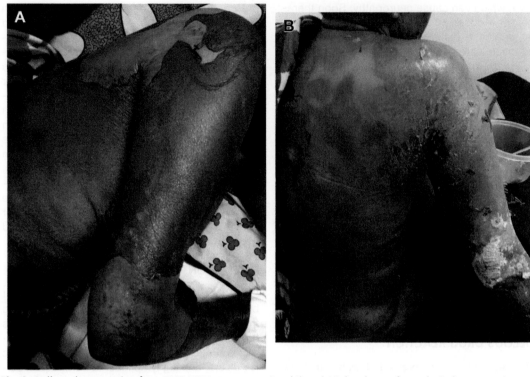

Fig. 6. Bullous drug reaction from TMP-SMX at presentation (*A*) and 10 days later after culprit drug cessation and skin-directed therapy using the bandages as protective dressings, without compression (*B*).

care treatment for these conditions. As traumatic injuries lead to disruption in lymphatic and venous blood vessels, it is not surprising that compression therapy would help to heal traumatic ulcers. For neuropathic ulcers and bullous drug eruptions, the bandages are used without compression to provide a protective dressing. For neuropathic ulcers, there is potentially the added benefit of offloading pressure that may be playing a role in the healing process. Of note, this case series is limited by the selection of cases from a range of clinical conditions that had positive outcomes, and there may be instances in which patients do not improve with this intervention. To evaluate the efficacy of these low-cost bandages, longitudinal studies with standardized and validated outcome measures for each disease of interest are required. A randomized controlled trial to assess the impact of these low-cost compression bandages on KS lymphedema is currently ongoing.[25]

In our experience, 2-component compression therapy is associated with few adverse events (eg, discomfort, itch) when used in an appropriate patient with an appropriate amount of compression. We consider compression therapy contraindicated in patients with a history of peripheral arterial disease or signs of peripheral arterial disease on examination (eg, cool limbs, poor distal pulses), untreated deep vein thrombosis, decompensated heart failure, and neuropathic ulcers. In the absence of reliable access to ankle-brachial index/toe-brachial index measurements and vascular imaging studies, physical examination findings are heavily relied on. Doppler ultrasound to evaluate for deep vein thrombosis is available in our setting. Compression bandages are applied weekly in clinic. This is consistent with standard of care practice around the world for 2-component compression therapy. Patients tend to have varying levels of tolerance for compression therapy and are counseled on potential for discomfort or pain. If the patient reports pain after application of the compression bandage, we reassess for contraindications, decrease the amount of compression by loosening the bandages, and recommend paracetamol (acetaminophen). We are unable to measure the exact amount of compression delivered because of the cost of interface pressure sensors. If pain persists, then compression therapy is aborted. Patients are instructed to call their provider if they develop pain after leaving the clinic, so that the provider can determine if the bandages should be removed and/or the patient should return to clinic sooner than previously planned. Because zinc oxide is inert and the only ingredient impregnated in the gauze, we would not expect to see allergic or irritant contact dermatitis; however, when patients are unable to keep the bandages dry because of the rainy season or their occupation (farming, fishing), pruritus does occur and can be associated with irritant contact dermatitis. This resolves with application of clean, dry bandages. During the rainy seasons, bandages are often changed more frequently, approximately every 3 days compared with every 7 days.

To-date, successful implementation of locally made bandages has been enabled by strong interdisciplinary collaboration among dermatology, pharmacy, oncology, and nursing. This collaboration has been fostered by the shared vision of addressing a commonly neglected group of skin conditions—wounds and lymphedema—that impact individuals, families, and their communities. From dermatology, oncology, pharmacy, and nursing, there are highly motivated individuals ("champions") who are collaborating members on the team. As providers managing wounds and lymphedema in Western Kenya are few and far between, our dermatologist and wound care nursing team members have appreciated exchange of ideas and clinical support from one another when faced with challenging cases and limited resources. Our pharmacy team members have been pivotal in helping to meet the increased demand for the bandages from the Fracture Clinic and have continued to maintain bandage supplies across multiple facilities. With more than a decade of partnership between the AMPATH revolving fund pharmacy and MOH pharmacies throughout Western Kenya,[21] the supply chain for bandage distribution was already in place, enabling efficient and timely delivery to health facilities.

From project inception, our primary objective was to support and train Kenyan providers in taking care of patients with wound and lymphedema care needs. Our project first began as a partnership between dermatology and pharmacy. With pilot grant funding, this grew to include oncology, with a focus on addressing the lymphedema care needs of patients with Kaposi sarcoma who are primarily treated at a subcounty health facility 3 hours away from MTRH. As patients with Kaposi sarcoma lymphedema began reporting improvement with symptoms and functioning associated with compression bandage use, our Kenyan team member began receiving referrals for patients with chronic wounds. The North America–based dermatology team was able to provide clinical mentorship through in-person meetings several times a year, coupled with remote mentorship via regular conference calls, WhatsApp messaging, and electronic mail communications.

This Kenyan team member now participates as a lead trainer in our wound and lymphedema care training sessions at other sites across Western Kenya.

Colleagues also introduced us to the MTRH Wound Clinic, directed by a nurse with specialized training in wound care. This nurse was eager, motivated, and qualified to develop wound care in both the outpatient and inpatient settings. The MTRH Wound Clinic is physically located next to the Fracture Clinic (Orthopedics) and, through successful healing of traumatic skin wounds associated with orthopedic injuries, there was a subsequent rise in awareness and popularity of the locally made low-cost bandages. In fact, from June 2018 through September 2019, 21 (37%) of 57 patients seen at the MTRH Wound Clinic had a traumatic skin wound associated with a fracture. Through partnership with nursing, we have been able to think more broadly and identify strategies for improving wound care across MTRH and Western Kenya. This increase in local capacity has enabled us to continue expanding access to additional patients.

For many patients in Western Kenya, weekly to twice weekly travel to MTRH, a national referral hospital, is not feasible because of time, transportation costs, lost income, and employment considerations. As such, increasing wound and lymphedema care capacity at county and sub-county health facilities that are referring patients to MTRH is needed. We have conducted several training sessions at a county facility where there is a high burden of chronic leg wounds, and nurses were keen on learning how to care for wounds with local resources. Our initial training session was open to everyone working at the facility. This was then followed by 2 sessions with a smaller group of nurses from sites throughout the facility who were interested in obtaining wound care training. We also conducted a training session at a sub-county facility where patients with Kaposi sarcoma receive care, with the goal of expanding facility-wide awareness of the uses of the bandages beyond Kaposi sarcoma lymphedema.

Moving forward, we will continue to train interested, motivated nurses and clinicians to provide wound and lymphedema care with local resources. Beyond training, we aim to support the development of wound care services at county/subcounty facilities. Ideally, a wound or lymphedema care "champion" would be identified at each of these health facilities to take leadership in this clinical domain, provide clinical support to lower-level health facilities, and appropriately refer to the national referral hospital level. Ongoing support can be provided through periodic training sessions, as well as telemedicine. Store-and-forward, asynchronous telemedicine would enable wound and lymphedema care providers to submit challenging cases to obtain guidance on diagnosis and management, which may include referral to MTRH for more specialized care.

Still, we need options for patients who cannot consistently access a health facility that has wound and lymphedema care capacity. In select patients, we have had success with training family members to perform wound/lymphedema care and apply the bandages, as described in the venous stasis ulcer case. For lymphedema from Kaposi sarcoma, some patients have performed self-care at home, including wrapping their own legs with the bandages. Home-based care delivery models, in which the patient or a caregiver assesses the wound and/or lymphedema and then applies the bandages as appropriate, is a promising option. Self-care and home-based care models have been successful for lymphedema from lymphatic filariasis,[26–30] podoconiosis,[31,32] and cancer.[27,33] In low-income and middle-income countries, self-bandaging for lymphedema from lymphatic filariasis[29] and podoconiosis[31,32] has been included in home-based care models. Evaluation of this approach and determination of optimal candidates for home-based care, as well as development of standardized training and assessment protocols, are needed in our setting. There are also opportunities to integrate the use of other materials into home-based care. For example, banana leaves have been used successfully for management of wounds,[34–36] with steam used as a sterilization technique.[36]

In sum, this project has made 2-component compression bandages affordable and more available to patients in Western Kenya. Since implementation, these bandages have been used with compression to treat venous leg ulcers, traumatic leg ulcers, and Kaposi sarcoma lymphedema, as well as without compression to treat neuropathic ulcers and bullous drug eruptions. Implementation of wound and lymphedema care has prioritized support and mentorship of Kenyan providers. Future studies should evaluate the efficacy of the locally made bandages in the treatment of venous leg ulcers, traumatic leg ulcers, lymphedema, neuropathic ulcers, and bullous drug eruptions. We have also made gains with improving utilization of these bandages at MTRH; however, there is imperative need to expand utilization to a much larger catchment area in Western Kenya. As Kenya has prioritized attainment of universal health coverage,[37] we must account for the various challenges that patients, families, and communities, as well as providers, health facilities, and health systems, face when providing care to an entire population.

ACKNOWLEDGMENTS

This project was supported, in part, with support from the Indiana Clinical and Translational Sciences Institute funded, in part by Grant Number UL1TR001108 from the National Institutes of Health (NIH), National Center for Advancing Translational Sciences, Clinical and Translational Sciences Award. Aileen Chang was supported by NIH Research Training Grant R25 TW009343 funded by the Fogarty International Center; the National Institute of Mental Health; the National Heart, Lung, and Blood Institute; and the Office of Research on Women's Health, as well as the University of California Global Health Institute (UCGHI). Sarah Coates is supported by the National Cancer Institute and the Fogarty International Center of NIH under Award Number D43TW009343, as well as UCGHI. The content is solely the responsibility of the authors and does not necessarily represent the official views of NIH or UCGHI. This project also received support from the Purdue University Office of Engagement and the American Academy of Dermatology's SkinCare for Developing Countries grant.

DISCLOSURE

The authors have nothing to disclose.

REFERENCES

1. Harrison MB, Graham ID, Friedberg E, et al. Regional planning study. Assessing the population with leg and foot ulcers. Can Nurse 2001;97(2):18–23.
2. Chokotho L, Mulwafu W, Jacobsen KH, et al. The burden of trauma in four rural district hospitals in Malawi: a retrospective review of medical records. Injury 2014;45(12):2065–70.
3. Sanyang E, Peek-Asa C, Bass P, et al. Injury factors associated with discharge status from emergency room at two major trauma hospitals in The Gambia, Africa. Injury 2017;48(7):1451–8.
4. Hulme P. Mechanisms of trauma at a rural hospital in Uganda. Pan Afr Med J 2010;7:5.
5. Ogendi JO, Ayisi JG. Causes of injuries resulting in a visit to the emergency department of a Provincial General Hospital, Nyanza, western Kenya. Afr Health Sci 2011;11(2):255–61.
6. Mousley E, Deribe K, Tamiru A, et al. Mental distress and podoconiosis in Northern Ethiopia: a comparative cross-sectional study. Int Health 2015;7(1):16–25.

7. Obindo J, Abdulmalik J, Nwefoh E, et al. Prevalence of depression and associated clinical and socio-demographic factors in people living with lymphatic filariasis in Plateau State, Nigeria. PLoS Negl Trop Dis 2017;11(6):e0005567.

8. Ton TG, Mackenzie C, Molyneux DH. The burden of mental health in lymphatic filariasis. Infect Dis Poverty 2015;4:34.

9. Abdulmalik J, Nwefoh E, Obindo J, et al. Emotional difficulties and experiences of stigma among persons with lymphatic filariasis in Plateau State, Nigeria. Health Hum Rights 2018;20(1):27–40.

10. Tora A, Mengiste A, Davey G, et al. Community involvement in the care of persons affected by podoconiosis-a lesson for other skin NTDs. Trop Med Infect Dis 2018;3(3):87.

11. Franks PJ, Moffatt CJ, Doherty DC, et al. Assessment of health-related quality of life in patients with lymphedema of the lower limb. Wound Repair Regen 2006;14(2):110–8.

12. Stolldorf DP, Dietrich MS, Ridner SH. A comparison of the quality of life in patients with primary and secondary lower limb lymphedema: a mixed-methods study. West J Nurs Res 2016;38(10):1313–34.

13. Babu BV, Swain BK, Rath K. Impact of chronic lymphatic filariasis on quantity and quality of productive work among weavers in an endemic village from India. Trop Med Int Health 2006;11(5):712–7.

14. Ramaiah KD, Das PK, Michael E, et al. The economic burden of lymphatic filariasis in India. Parasitol Today 2000;16(6):251–3.

15. Ramaiah KD, Guyatt H, Ramu K, et al. Treatment costs and loss of work time to individuals with chronic lymphatic filariasis in rural communities in south India. Trop Med Int Health 1999;4(1):19–25.

16. Ramaiah KD, Radhamani MP, John KR, et al. The impact of lymphatic filariasis on labour inputs in southern India: results of a multi-site study. Ann Trop Med Parasitol 2000;94(4):353–64.

17. Tekola F, Mariam DH, Davey G. Economic costs of endemic non-filarial elephantiasis in Wolaita Zone, Ethiopia. Trop Med Int Health 2006;11(7):1136–44.

18. Grada AA, Phillips TJ. Lymphedema: diagnostic workup and management. J Am Acad Dermatol 2017;77(6):995–1006.

19. O'Meara S, Cullum N, Nelson EA, et al. Compression for venous leg ulcers. Cochrane Database Syst Rev 2012;(11):CD000265.

20. Chang AY, Tonui EC, Momanyi D, et al. Development of low-cost locally sourced two-component compression bandages in Western Kenya. Dermatol Ther (Heidelb) 2018;8(3):475–81.

21. Manji I, Manyara SM, Jakait B, et al. The Revolving Fund Pharmacy Model: backing up the Ministry of Health supply chain in western Kenya. Int J Pharm Pract 2016;24(5):358–66.

22. Lyvers E, Elliott DP. Topical metronidazole for odor control in pressure ulcers. Consult Pharm 2015;30(9):523–6.

23. Paul JC, Pieper BA. Topical metronidazole for the treatment of wound odor: a review of the literature. Ostomy Wound Manage 2008;54(3):18–27 [quiz 28–9].

24. Campisi C, Boccardo F. Microsurgical techniques for lymphedema treatment: derivative lymphatic-venous microsurgery. World J Surg 2004;28(6):609–13.

25. Chang AY, Karwa R, Busakhala N, et al. Randomized controlled trial to evaluate locally sourced two-component compression bandages for HIV-associated Kaposi sarcoma leg lymphedema in western Kenya: The Kenyan Improvised Compression for Kaposi Sarcoma (KICKS) study protocol. Contemp Clin Trials Commun 2018;12:116–22.

26. Aggithaya MG, Narahari SR, Vayalil S, et al. Self care integrative treatment demonstrated in rural community setting improves health related quality of life of lymphatic filariasis patients in endemic villages. Acta Trop 2013;126(3):198–204.

27. Douglass J, Graves P, Gordon S. Self-care for management of secondary lymphedema: a systematic review. PLoS Negl Trop Dis 2016;10(6):e0004740.

28. Jullien P, Some J, Brantus P, et al. Efficacy of home-based lymphoedema management in reducing acute attacks in subjects with lymphatic filariasis in Burkina Faso. Acta Trop 2011;120(Suppl 1):S55–61.

29. Narahari SR, Bose KS, Aggithaya MG, et al. Community level morbidity control of lymphoedema using self care and integrative treatment in two lymphatic filariasis endemic districts of South India: a non randomized interventional study. Trans R Soc Trop Med Hyg 2013;107(9):566–77.

30. Wijesinghe RS, Wickremasinghe AR, Ekanayake S, et al. Efficacy of a limb-care regime in preventing acute adenolymphangitis in patients with lymphoedema caused by bancroftian filariasis, in Colombo, Sri Lanka. Ann Trop Med Parasitol 2007;101(6):487–97.

31. Negussie H, Kassahun MM, Fegan G, et al. Podoconiosis treatment in northern Ethiopia (GoLBet): study protocol for a randomised controlled trial. Trials 2015;16:307.

32. Negussie H, Molla M, Ngari M, et al. Lymphoedema management to prevent acute dermatolymphangioadenitis in podoconiosis in northern Ethiopia (GoLBeT): a pragmatic randomised controlled trial. Lancet Glob Health 2018;6(7):e795–803.

33. Ridner SH, Fu MR, Wanchai A, et al. Self-manage-
ment of lymphedema: a systematic review of the
literature from 2004 to 2011. Nurs Res 2012;61(4):
291–9.

34. Bitter CC, Erickson TB. Management of burn injuries
in the wilderness: lessons from low-resource settings. Wilderness Environ Med 2016;27(4):519–25.

35. Gore MA, Akolekar D. Evaluation of banana leaf
dressing for partial thickness burn wounds. Burns
2003;29(5):487–92.

36. Guenova E, Hoetzenecker W, Kisuze G, et al. Banana leaves as an alternative wound dressing.
Dermatol Surg 2013;39(2):290–7.

37. Kenya Ministry of Health. Transforming Health:
Accelerating Attainment of Universal Health
Coverage. Kenya Health Sector Strategic and Investment Plan (KHSSPI), July 2013-June 2017.
Available at: https://www.who.int/pmnch/media/
events/2013/kenya_hssp.pdf. Accessed January 9,
2020.

Neglected Populations

Challenges of Managing Skin Diseases in Refugees and Migrants

Valeska Padovese, MD[a],*, Alexia Knapp, MD[b]

KEYWORDS

- Skin disease • Dermatology • Sexually transmitted infections • HIV • Refugee • Asylum seeker
- Migrant • Internally displaced person

KEY POINTS

- Providing skin care to displaced populations might pose significant challenges related to the pattern of migration, availability of trained health providers, and limited formularies.
- Skin diseases in migrants encompass communicable and noncommunicable diseases. Health providers should be trained to recognize skin signs of torture and to deal with cultural-related issues.
- Immunization, hygiene, and sanitation, including access to food and clean water, have an impact on skin health and might cause infectious disease outbreaks in the camps.
- Screening policies in migrant populations are not standardized across different countries, posing challenges in early detection and prevention of communicable diseases.

INTRODUCTION

Currently an unprecedented 70.8 million individuals worldwide are forcibly displaced from their homes because of war, violence, and persecution.[1] Among these are 25.9 million refugees, 41.3 million internally displaced persons (IDPs), and 3.5 million persons seeking asylum.[1] These figures do not include migrants who may be leaving their homes because of poverty to seek better economic opportunities or those fleeing natural disasters or adverse environmental conditions due to climate change. There is a high prevalence of skin diseases among displaced populations due to multiple factors related to the stress of displacement and forced migration. These include overcrowding, exposure to the elements, food insecurity, and breakdown of health care infrastructure. There are numerous challenges in management of skin diseases in displaced

populations because of lack of reliable information pertaining to the epidemiology of skin diseases, few trained dermatology specialists working in these settings, and limited diagnostic and therapeutic resources in refugee camps.

DEFINITIONS PERTAINING TO DISPLACED INDIVIDUALS

There are several terms to describe displaced individuals and populations, including refugee,[2,3] IDP,[4] person seeking asylum (asylum seeker, asylee),[5] and migrant[2] (**Table 1**). The term refugee is a legal definition and has implications pertaining to protection under international law. The terms refugee and migrant are not synonymous, although migrants may still need humanitarian assistance.[2,6]

[a] Genitourinary Clinic, Department of Dermatology and Venereology, Mater Dei Hospital, International Foundation for Dermatology Migrant Health Dermatology Working Group, GU Clinic, Mater Dei Hospital, Triq Dun Karm, L-Imsida, MSD2090, Malta; [b] Department of Dermatology, HealthPartners Medical Group, International Foundation for Dermatology Migrant Health Dermatology Working Group, 401 Phalen Boulevard, Mailstop 41102B, Saint Paul, MN 55130, USA
* Corresponding author.
E-mail address: valeska.padovese@gov.mt

Dermatol Clin 39 (2021) 101–115
https://doi.org/10.1016/j.det.2020.08.010

Table 1
Summary of definitions

Refugee	• A person unwilling or unable to return to his or her country of nationality because of persecution or well-founded fear of persecution due to race, religion, nationality, membership in a particular social group, or political opinion • By definition has crossed an international border • Protected status under international law
Internally displaced person	• A person fleeing persecution or violence, but within the borders of country of origin • Among the most vulnerable of displaced people • May reside in a protection of civilians (POC) camp
Person seeking asylum (asylum seeker; asylee)	• An individual formally seeking protection in another country whose request has not yet been processed • Reasons for seeking asylum include unwillingness or inability to return to their country of nationality because of persecution or well-founded fear of persecution due to race, religion, nationality, membership in a particular social group, or political opinion • If asylum is granted, the asylee's status changes to refugee
Migrant, international migrant	• Person who has moved from his or her habitual place of residence regardless of the reason for migration or legal status • Temporary or permanent basis • Not a formal legal definition • Not synonymous with refugee • Migrants may still need humanitarian assistance and are protected by international human rights law • Subcategories include economic migrant, irregular or undocumented migrant

BARRIERS TO PROVIDING DERMATOLOGIC CARE

There are immense challenges to providing dermatologic care to displaced populations. The large number of affected people, their movement within and across international borders, armed conflict that impacts security and access to resources,[7] limited access to dermatology expertise, and lack of therapeutic options all pose barriers to managing skin diseases in these populations.

Approximately 80% of refugees are hosted in neighboring countries, which are predominantly low and middle income (LMIC).[1] According to United Nations High Commissioner for Refugees (UNHCR), 2.6 million refugees live in camps, whereas the remaining majority live in urban areas or informal settlements.[8] The largest refugee camps are located in Bangladesh, Uganda, Kenya, Jordan, Tanzania, and Ethiopia.[8] UNHCR-sponsored refugee camps are intended to provide safety, security, medical care, legal advice, and temporary shelter for refugees.[8] Refugees may live in camps for months to several years in protracted refugee situations.[9] During emergent humanitarian crises, UNHCR prioritizes the following health interventions: providing primary care, decreasing morbidity due to epidemics, improving childhood survival, prevention and control of noncommunicable disease, rational access to specialist care, and integration into national health services.[10] Implementation of water, sanitation, hygiene measures, and nutrition services is closely integrated into its public health strategy in refugee camps. Medical care in refugee camps is typically provided in partnership with nongovernmental organizations and/or the national health care systems in host countries.

Few studies in the peer-reviewed literature address the epidemiology of skin diseases in refugee and migrant populations (**Box 1**). The prevalence of skin diseases appears to be high, ranging from 18.7% to 96.2%,[11–15] depending on the population evaluated and geographic region. Dermatologic disorders are sometimes grouped as "disorder of the skin and subcutaneous tissue" without further differentiation.[15] Dermatitis and infectious dermatoses, especially bacterial and fungal infections and scabies, are among the most commonly observed diagnoses (**Table 2**).[12–14]

Box 1
What is the literature lacking?

- Epidemiology of skin diseases among refugees, migrants, internally displaced persons
- Best practices for diagnosis and management of skin diseases in displaced populations
- Determinants of skin health in displaced populations

With resources mainly allocated to basic medical care in humanitarian crises, there is limited diagnostic testing available for dermatologic disorders and most diagnoses are made clinically.[14,16] In addition, medications available for management of cutaneous disorders are restricted. Outlined in **Table 3** is the essential drug formulary for Médecins Sans Frontières (MSF; Doctors Without Borders) which lists only hydrocortisone 1% cream and ointment as topical anti-inflammatory medications.[17] The World Health Organization Model List of Essential Medicines includes betamethasone valerate 0.1% cream or ointment in addition to 1% hydrocortisone.[18] By comparison, a recent report of a field-mission assessment of Syrian refugees in Jordan had similar topical medications available, with a few additional options for topical corticosteroids.[16]

ENVIRONMENTAL EXPOSURES AFFECTING THE SKIN OF MIGRANTS IN TRANSIT, AT ARRIVAL, AND IN CAMPS

The health of displaced persons is affected by the conditions during travel and the living conditions in the receiving country. Thousands of migrants cross the Mediterranean Sea by boat every year, often using overcrowded, uncovered small boats. The journey lasts several days, during which migrants are exposed to extreme conditions, including cold or hot weather, precipitation, deficient hygiene, inadequate food and water, prolonged sitting in the same position and immersion of feet in contaminated sea water. Dermatologic conditions observed at arrival of sea migrants are therefore related to this perilous sea crossing. Skin diseases commonly seen at migrants' arrival by boat in the Southern Mediterranean region include scabies, secondary bacterial infections, bacterial cellulitis, deep abscesses, and tissue necrosis[19,20] (**Fig 1**). An unusual skin and soft tissue infection of the lower limbs known as "Patera foot" (named after small fishing boats called "pateras" used for the sea crossing) has been described in otherwise young, healthy migrants traveling by sea from sub-Saharan Africa. Patera foot occurs in the setting of prolonged immobilization and immersion of feet in water contaminated by urine, decaying food, or fuel.[19]

Irritant dermatitis due to extended contact with sea water and sunburn are commonly seen in summer. Hypothermia, cold water injuries, and frostbite occur during the winter. Chemical burns, usually on the buttocks and posterior thighs, result from prolonged contact with a mix of sea water, petrol, and urine. There are reports of scald burns of the hands and upper arms from accidently touching the boat engine or by self-infliction, when asylum seekers attempt to obliterate their fingerprints at arrival in order to be relocated to a different country (**Fig 2**).

Plantar callouses, keratoderma, and infected wounds secondary to ruptured friction blisters have been observed in Syrian and Afghani refugees walking barefoot or wearing inappropriate shoes during extended journeys on foot. Trauma-related injuries are among the most common issues facing the Syrian refugees at arrival in the Eastern Greek islands.[21] For young, otherwise healthy migrants, the transit period may have no health consequences because of the short duration. For others, such as those experiencing trafficking or smuggling as a means of arrival or who remain in detention centers, the transition period can greatly affect health. Detention centers for migrants reduce access to health care. In Morocco, nearly half of all MSF medical visits in 2012 were related to poor social and living conditions due to insecure travel routes and precarious settlements.[21] Forced migration exposes individuals to socioeconomic, cultural, and environmental changes; therefore, initial healthiness can be undermined by difficult living conditions on arrival.

MALNUTRITION

In the context of forced migration and food insecurity, malnutrition is a significant concern for refugees, especially in children who may suffer from growth stunting and cognitive impairment. The World Health Organization defines childhood global acute malnutrition (GAM) and severe acute malnutrition (SAM) with weight-for-height z scores or mid-upper arm circumference[22] (**Table 4**) and sets a threshold of 15% prevalence of GAM in global emergencies. In a recent study, the prevalence of GAM among Rohingya refugee children aged 6 to 59 months was 24.3% and the prevalence of chronic malnutrition was 43.4.%.[23]

Table 2
Epidemiology of skin diseases in refugees and migrants

Setting	Demographics	Skin Diseases Reported
Al Za'atari Refugee Camp and Jordanian towns near the Syrian border • Saikal et al. JEADV 2020[16]	288 patients 37.9% male 84.0% from Syria 15.9% from Jordan	• Inflammatory diseases (71.9%) ○ Dermatitis/eczema (33.8%) ○ Disorders of skin appendages (12.7%) ○ Other disorders of skin and subcutaneous tissue (15.1%) ○ Papulosquamous disorders (6.9%) ○ Urticaria and erythema (2.4%) ○ Radiation-related disorders of the skin (0.6%) • Infectious and parasitic skin diseases (20.8%) ○ Fungal infection (7.9%) ○ Viral infection (8.5%) ○ Bacterial infection (3.2%) ○ Pediculosis, ascariasis, and other infestations (1.2%) ○ Protozoal infection (0%) • Other conditions (7.9%) ○ Neoplasms (3.0%) ○ Diseases of the circulatory system (2.7%) ○ Injury, poisoning (0.6%) ○ Others (1.5%)
Rural Nyala, Sudan, 12 orphanages, and 2 refugee camps • Kibal Ozturk, IJD 2019[14]	1802 patients • 1182 from orphanages and refugee camps (ORC) • 620 from community outreach clinics (OC) Age range 2–72 y; Mean 24 ± 9.33 y (ORC) 1–95 y; Mean 27 ± 8.14 y (OC)	• 92.6% of persons examined had skin disease • Fungal infections most common (32.6%) • Dermatitis/eczema (10.5%) • Bacterial skin infections (10.3%) • Disorders of skin appendages (8.7%) • Disorders of pigmentation (7.4%) • Hypertrophic skin disorders (6.4%) • Viral infections (5.8%) • Benign neoplasm (1.9%) • Dermatoses due to animal injury (0.4%) • Bullous dermatoses (0.1%) • Malignant neoplasms (0.1%)

(continued on next page)

Table 2
(continued)

Setting	Demographics	Skin Diseases Reported
Migrants arriving on the Italian coast Di Meco, Eur J Public Health 2018[13]	7946 migrants 83.5% male Mean age 21.6 y (±7.3 y) Most from Eritrea, Nigeria, Somalia	• Scabies (58%) • Skin and soft tissue infections (10.3%) • Itch (8.9%) • Pediculosis (8.8%) • Dermatitis (7.5%) • Varicella (2.3%) • Insect bites (2.0%) • Burns (1.5%) • Skin mycoses (1.4%) • Herpes simplex virus (0.4%)
Migrants living in Maltese reception centers Padovese, Eur J Public Health 2013[12]	2216 migrants 82.7% male Mean age 25 y 70.1% from Somalia	• 21.9% with skin disease • Contact dermatitis and other eczema (13.0%) • Pruritus (11.6%) • Scar (9.5%) • Scabies (8.2%) • Acne (8.2%) • Pityriasis versicolor (7.3%) • Others (42.2%) • 1 case of multibacillary leprosy

Data from Refs.[12–14,16]

Table 3
Topical medications available in refugee camps

Drug Class	Médecins Sans Frontières Essential Drug Formulary	Al Za'atari Refugee Camp

Antifungal	Miconazole 2% cream
	Whitfield ointment
	  (benzoic acid + salicylic acid)
		Terbinafine 1% cream
		Ketoconazole 1% shampoo
		Whitfield ointment
		  (benzoic acid + salicylic acid)

Antibacterial	Mupirocin 2% ointment Silver sulfadiazine 1% cream	Clindamycin 1% gel
Scabicides	Benzyl benzoate 25% lotion Permethrin 5% cream	Benzyl benzoate 25% lotion
Pediculicides	Permethrin 1% lotion Malathion 0.5% lotion	
Antiseptics	Chlorhexidine Povidone iodine	

Topical corticosteroids	Hydrocortisone 1% cream
	  and ointment
		Clobetasol propionate 0.05%
		Mometasone furoate 0.1%
		Hydrocortisone 1%
		Combined preparation:
		  triamcinolone, neomycin, nystatin

Antipruritic	Calamine lotion 8 or 15% lotion	
Emollient	Petroleum jelly	Petroleum jelly
Antimitotic/antiviral	Podophyllotoxin 0.5% solution	

Data from Saikal, S.L., et al., Skin disease profile of Syrian refugees in Jordan: a field-mission assessment. J Eur Acad Dermatol Venereol, 2020. 34(2): p. 419-425. And MSF Medical Guidelines, Essential Drugs. Drugs for external use, antiseptics and disinfectants. [cited 2020 January 25]; Available from: https://medicalguidelines.msf.org/viewport/EssDr/english/drugs-for-external-use-antiseptics-and-disinfectants-16688511.html.

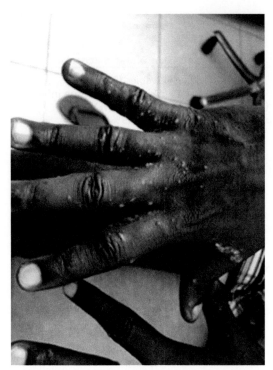

Fig. 1. Scabies with secondary bacterial infection on the hands in a boat migrant after arrival in Malta.

Cutaneous signs of SAM include bilateral pitting edema, generalized desquamation, hyperpigmentation or hypopigmentation, and alopecia. Systemic manifestations include loss of muscle mass, enlarged abdomen, fatigue, irritability, and increased susceptibility to infections.

Micronutrient deficiencies occur in displaced populations where food insecurity exists or in populations dependent on food aid. Not all

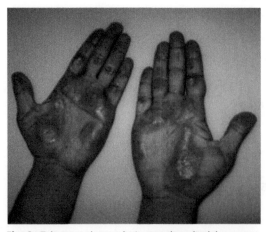

Fig. 2. Eritrean migrant in Lampedusa (Italy) presenting with a scald injury of the palmar aspects of hands caused by contact with the boat engine.

micronutrient deficiencies cause clinical symptoms. There is no single solution to prevent micronutrient deficiencies, so a multifaceted interventional approach involving fortification of relief food, supplementation, extra rations for trade, and promotion of kitchen gardens is recommended[24–27] (**Table 5**).

INFECTIOUS DISEASES BURDEN AND NEGLECTED TROPICAL DISEASES IN REFUGEES AND MIGRANTS: EPIDEMIOLOGIC BRIDGING AND BARRIERS TO ACCESS OF HEALTH SERVICES

The primary determinant of infectious disease risk in displaced persons on arrival is the epidemiology of infectious diseases in their countries of origin.[28] The epidemiologic bridging produced by migration is directly related to the degree of difference between origin and destination, and to the size of the mobile population that moves between the different disease prevalence patterns.[29] The conditions of the migration journey and access to health services at arrival and post migration impact health. However, it is important to recognize the heterogeneous nature of refugee and migrant groups. Even migrant groups with good access to health care may still be at risk for preventable and treatable infectious diseases.[30] Differing patterns of migration may impact the infectious disease risk and burden in migrants. Irregular migration is associated with precarious journeys and increases the risk of exposure to violence, trafficking, crowded living conditions, and transmission of infections through direct contact, blood, and airborne routes. Regular migration with planned movement has a lower risk of infectious disease exposures during transit than irregular migration irrespective of whether the migration is forced (refugees) or nonforced (economic migrants).[31,32]

The increased migratory flux through the Mediterranean route during the past few years, especially from sub-Saharan Africa, has led to an increased number of individuals affected by neglected tropical diseases (NTDs) in Mediterranean countries. A survey focused on NTD cases (schistosomiasis, strongyloidiasis, cystic echinococcosis, Chagas disease, leishmaniasis, cysticercosis, filariasis, and scabies) conducted in 9 infectious and tropical diseases sentinel centers in Italy in a 7-year period reported that 69% of the NTDs diagnosed were in foreign-born subjects, mainly strongyloidiasis and schistosomiasis.[33,34] The European Center for Disease Prevention and Control recommends screening using antibody-detecting serologic tests and

Table 4
Nutritional status measurement in protracted refugee situations

WHO definitions of malnutrition	Weight-for-Height/ Length z Score	Mid-upper Arm Circumference, mm	Height/Length-For-Age z Score
Global acute malnutrition (GAM)	<−2	<125	
Severe acute malnutrition (SAM)	<−3	<115	
Chronic malnutrition			<−2

treatment for schistosomiasis and strongyloidiasis in migrants from endemic countries.[35]

Although scabies is commonly diagnosed in migrants, there are no recommendations for screening and mass drug administration. Scabies lesions are often secondarily infected with the bacteria *Streptococcus pyogenes* or *Staphylococcus aureus,* which can cause local skin infections such as impetigo and cellulitis. Streptococcal infection can lead to septicemia and postinfection complications, including end-stage renal failure and acute rheumatic fever. Ivermectin mass drug administration to control scabies in asylum seekers has been shown to be feasible and effective, with reduced risk of re-infestations and complications.[36]

Cutaneous leishmaniasis (CL) is the most prevalent NTD in the conflict zone in the Middle East. Ongoing civil war in Syria has resulted in the mass migration of 5 million Syrians to neighboring countries, and this has led to increased CL prevalence and possible local transmission by indigenous sandflies. Outbreaks of CL among Syrian refugees have been reported in Lebanon[37] and Jordan,[38] previously low-prevalence countries (**Fig 3**). Molecular diagnosis of imported CL cases in Syrian refugees and migrants in Turkey indicates the changing epidemiologic features of CL in the region. This includes a case of *Leishmaniasis aethiopica* infection detected in a Syrian refugee in Turkey who never traveled outside the country, meaning that there might be a focus or multiple foci of infection in Syria as well as a suitable vector and reservoir.[39]

Migrants traveling back to their country of origin are at increased risk for infectious diseases because they do not seek pretravel medical advice and adopt local behaviors while visiting their home country. On return, infectious diseases that disproportionately affect this population include malaria, vaccine-preventable diseases, hepatitis A and B, tuberculosis, and sexually transmitted infections.[28,30]

VACCINE-PREVENTABLE COMMUNICABLE DISEASES WITH MUCOCUTANEOUS MANIFESTATIONS

Vaccine-preventable diseases (VPDs) occur in humanitarian emergencies due to overcrowding, malnutrition, poor sanitation, and breakdown in the health care systems that provide routine immunizations.[40] VPDs in displaced populations include measles, polio, hepatitis A, meningococcal meningitis, cholera, yellow fever,[40] and varicella.[41] Refugees being resettled to a third country, such as the United States, are immunized against measles and varicella before departure, depending on age.[42]

Measles

Measles is a highly contagious, vaccine-preventable respiratory disease caused by a paramyxovirus that is transmitted via droplet exposure. It causes high fever, morbilliform exanthem, conjunctivitis, and coryza. Complications include otitis media, pneumonia, encephalitis, and death. Measles mortality appears to be much higher in refugee settings.[43] Epidemics of measles have occurred in humanitarian crises driven by overcrowding and movement between camp environments and surrounding host communities[40] (**Box 2**). Therefore, measles immunization is prioritized in humanitarian crises (**Box 3**). A measles outbreak with more than 1700 cases occurred among Rohingya refugees in Cox's Bazar, Bangladesh, in September-November 2017.[44] The measles immunization rates for the Rohingya population was low before the outbreak.[44] A large-scale measles immunization campaign was implemented with almost 350,000 children immunized, approximately 96% coverage, which may have averted a larger outbreak.[44,45]

Varicella

Primary varicella (chickenpox) is a highly contagious infection caused by the varicella-zoster virus

Table 5
Micronutrient deficiencies with mucocutaneous manifestations

Micronutrient and Risk Factors for Deficiency	Clinical Manifestations of Deficiency	Reports of Deficiency in Humanitarian Crises	Population-Based Management Strategies to Reduce Micronutrient Deficiencies
Niacin (Vitamin B3) and/or tryptophan Higher risk of deficiency in populations consuming primarily maize (corn) and/or sorghum	• Pellagra • Photosensitive rash • Diarrhea • Dementia • Death	Mozambican refugees in Malawi (1989). Occurred when distribution of groundnuts ceased and were substituted with beans that required prolonged cooking. Bhutanese refugees in Nepal (1994). Diet mainly polished rice, perished vegetables. Pellagra, scurvy, beriberi observed.	Reintroduction of groundnuts to rations. Fortification of maize with niacin (van den Briel, 2007).[39] Micronutrient-enriched blended food (corn-soy blend).
Vitamin C Occurs in settings with prolonged inadequate access fresh produce Depletion of vitamin C stores in the body occurs in 2–3 mo	Scurvy Gingival swelling and/or bleeding Hyperkeratosis Corkscrew hairs Joint swelling and pain, especially of the lower limbs, which may interfere with ambulation Chest pain	Kakuma refugee camp, Kenya 2017–2018 (Ververs, 2019[75]). Young adult and adolescent male individuals. Previous scurvy outbreaks in Kakuma in 2003 and 1995–1997. Ethiopian refugees (Desenclos, 1989[71]; Seaman and Rivers, 1989[72]).	• Distribution of variety of fresh foods. • Vitamin supplementation. • Extra rations for trade. • Fortification of relief food. • Promotion of kitchen gardens. • Cultivation of produce that can be sold or traded. • Cash assistance to purchase produce.
Vitamin A Risk of deficiency in populations with poor dietary intake, including those dependent on food aid with inadequate levels of vitamin A	Night blindness Bitot spots on the conjunctiva Xerophthalmia Keratomalacia Increased morbidity and mortality from respiratory and gastrointestinal infections Dry skin, dry lips	Vitamin A deficiency (serum retinol) in 20.5%–61.7% of refugees in camps in Kenya, Uganda, Ethiopia, Algeria (Seal, 2005). Vitamin A deficiency in 6% of women and 28% of children in refugee camps on border of Jordan (Khatib, 2009[74]).	Maize meal fortification (Seal, 2008) resulted in decreased vitamin A deficiency in adolescents in Nangweshi refugee camp, Zambia.

(continued on next page)

Table 5 (continued)			
Micronutrient and Risk Factors for Deficiency	Clinical Manifestations of Deficiency	Reports of Deficiency in Humanitarian Crises	Population-Based Management Strategies to Reduce Micronutrient Deficiencies
Iron Risk of deficiency is higher among women of child-bearing age and children with poor dietary intake of iron and vitamin C	Anemia Fatigue Impaired childhood development Pallor	Anemia in 12.8%–72.9% of refugees in camps in Kenya, Uganda, Ethiopia, Algeria (Seal, 2005[73]). Anemia in 45% of women and 75% of children and iron deficiency in 44% of women and 64% of children in refugee camps on border with Jordan (Khatib, 2009[74]).	Maize meal fortification (Seal, 2008[27]) resulted in decreased anemia in children in Nangweshi refugee camp, Zambia.

Data from Refs.[24–27,71–75]

(Fig 4). It is transmitted via direct skin contact and inhalation of aerosolized vesicular fluid and respiratory secretions. In healthy children, this self-limited illness lasts 4 to 7 days and is characterized by a generalized pruritic vesicular eruption, fever, and malaise. Recovery from infection usually confers life-long immunity.[46] The risk of complications, such as secondary bacterial infection, pneumonia, and encephalitis is higher in infants, adults, pregnant women, and immunocompromised persons. Routine immunization to varicella is not included in most national vaccination programs.[47] High levels of natural immunity to varicella occur by adolescence for most individuals in temperate climates.[47] There appears to be a higher prevalence of seronegative adults from tropical regions.[48]

Varicella outbreaks have occurred in densely populated refugee camps, including a 2008 outbreak among Lao refugees in Thailand that affected 4% (309 of 7815) of the camp population.[41] A more recent epidemic of varicella occurred in Rohingya refugees in Bangladesh, affecting 59,172 people by March 2019.[49] Smaller varicella outbreaks have also been reported among 31 adult migrants primarily from Sudan and Eritrea in Calais, France,[50] and asylum

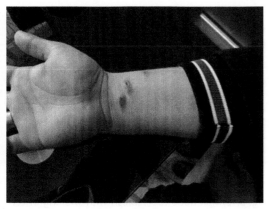

Fig. 3. CL in a Syrian refugee in Al Za'atari camp (Jordan).

Box 2
Factors contributing to outbreaks of measles in humanitarian crises[40,43]

- Lower vaccination rates (17%–57% of population) or only single dose of vaccine received
- Poor living conditions
- Movement of refugees
- Poor nutritional status
- Status and effectiveness of control measures

Data from Lam, E., A. McCarthy, and M. Brennan, Vaccine-preventable diseases in humanitarian emergencies among refugee and internally-displaced populations. Hum Vaccin Immunother, 2015. 11(11): p. 2627-36. And Kouadio, I.K., T. Kamigaki, and H. Oshitani, Measles outbreaks in displaced populations: a re-view of transmission, morbidity and mortality associated factors. BMC Int Health Hum Rights, 2010. 10:5.

seekers residing in a center in Italy.[51] Strategies to prevent outbreaks involve immunizing individuals with no prior history of varicella, including contacts of known cases,[52] isolation of cases, and appropriate management of acute zoster cases to prevent exposure of susceptible individuals to virus.[49]

TUBERCULOSIS, HUMAN IMMUNODEFICIENCY VIRUS, AND OTHER SEXUALLY TRANSMITTED INFECTIONS

Migrants in Europe face a disproportionate burden of tuberculosis (TB), human immunodeficiency virus (HIV), and hepatitis B and C. Overall, approximately 30% of TB cases in the European Union (EU) are in migrants, with considerable variation between countries. The key risk groups with the highest incidence and risk of active TB following migration are migrants from Asia and Africa, recent migrants (within 5 years of arrival), refugees, and individuals with comorbidities such as HIV infection or diabetes mellitus (**Fig 5**).

Hepatitis B prevalence in migrants in Europe is estimated to be 6 times higher and hepatitis C prevalence 2 times higher than the general population. Although migrants face the largest burden of infectious diseases in Europe, there is evidence that these disparities are attributable not only to higher prevalence in migrants' countries of origin, but also poor living conditions and barriers to health care in transit and host countries.[53]

The HIV epidemic in Europe is characterized by a disproportionate number of infections among migrants, with an estimated 37% of new HIV diagnoses acquired post migration. Migrants are usually late presenters, have poor HIV treatment outcomes, and are likely to transmit to contacts if undiagnosed. Access to HIV care remains a challenge in many European countries, which results in increased stigma and discrimination, discouragement from testing, and enhanced transmission. Sexually transmitted infections (STIs) are often increased in migrants with high-risk behaviors or due to sexual abuse during the transit phase. Contributing factors to STIs/HIV infection are social inequalities associated with migration (eg, low income, unemployment, poor housing),

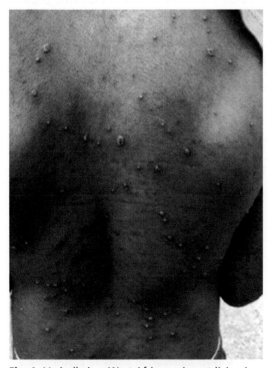

Fig. 4. Varicella in a West African migrant living in a reception center in Malta. A small outbreak was reported in October 2019.

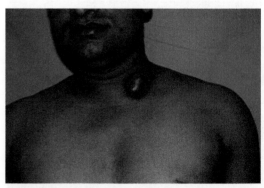

Fig. 5. Lymph node tuberculosis with swelling of cervical lymph nodes in a migrant from Bangladesh (INMP-Rome, Italy).

human trafficking, HIV-related stigma and discrimination, and changes in sexual behavior after migration.[54]

These findings support the efforts toward creating a common European standard for migrants' health testing at reception and during settlement; moreover, the expansion of testing beyond sexual health and antenatal settings is recommended. Testing opportunities should be linked with combination prevention measures such as access to pre-exposure prophylaxis and treatment as prevention of asylum seekers and refugees.[54,55]

SCREENING POLICIES IN MIGRANT POPULATIONS

Most screening in Europe focuses on active or latent TB infection and specifically targets asylum seekers and refugees. Australia, Canada, New Zealand, the United Kingdom, and the United States require prearrival screening and treatment for active TB for all immigrant applicants, including refugees who are resettling. These countries have variable requirements for screening for other infectious diseases, such as syphilis, HIV, and viral hepatitis.[56] The United States also has a comprehensive predeparture health assessment and treatment program for refugees in which vaccines are updated and presumptive treatment for intestinal parasites, schistosomiasis, and malaria treatment are given, depending on country of processing. Screening for leprosy, scabies, and pediculosis is also performed. This program has resulted in decreased burden of intestinal parasites after arrival and was found to be cost-effective.[56]

Recently, there has been renewed focus on incorporating latent TB screening into immigrant screening programs and exploring whether we need to additionally encompass diseases such as hepatitis and HIV. Cost-effectiveness of active screening has been debated because migrants with infections detected through active screening are more likely to experience shorter symptomatic periods, reduced infectious periods, and lower risk of hospital admission than those identified passively, pointing to the benefit of active screening. Five studies examining the acceptability of screening for HIV, hepatitis B and C, and TB identified that both migrants and service providers perceived the screenings to be acceptable.[56,57] Screening for HIV and hepatitis B and C is also recommended in reception camps but linkage to care and completion of vaccination may be challenging, especially in highly mobile irregular migrants.[57]

Screening for leprosy is cost-effective and should be recommended in migrants from endemic areas. Leprosy presents with skin manifestation or nerve enlargement in the early clinical phase, which can be successfully treated to prevent morbidity. Studies show that leprosy screening would detect about three-quarters of leprosy cases that could arise in the 10-year period post migration.[58] A comprehensive skin diseases screening at arrival and in the camps should include scabies, pediculosis, fungal infections, and according to the area of origin and endemicity, CL and leprosy. Flow charts and tables may support clinicians in the diagnostic process.

At arrival in the host country, a medical check-up based on a syndromic approach should be conducted to detect diseases of public health concern. Skin health assessment is recommended as part of this approach to facilitate early detection and to prevent transmission of scabies, pediculosis, and cutaneous fungal infections.[30]

TORTURE AND VIOLENCE
Torture: Management of Physical and Psychological Sequelae

Many refugees and asylum seekers, including children, have experienced torture. Worldwide, only approximately one-third of asylum applicants are granted protected status and ensured personal safety from repeated torture or death.[59] Common methods of torture include being burnt by cigarettes and having scalding hot liquids poured on the body. Blunt trauma includes punching, kicking, slapping, *falaka* (being beaten on the soles of the feet), and being assaulted with truncheons and wires.[59,60]

Dermatologists may be faced with patients with unique dermatologic findings, such as chemical weapon burns, rubber bullet contusions, and electrical shock injuries from primitive electrodes. Identification and documentation of physical injuries are critical for verifying the credibility of allegations in political asylum and torture survivors.[60] In addition, inadequate mental health care may result in undertreatment of severe psychological disorders, such as posttraumatic stress disorders. Health professionals are requested to identify and document injuries related to torture, despite very little specialized training to address this issue.[60]

Gender-based Violence

Female refugees and migrants face specific challenges, particularly in maternal, sexual, and reproductive health. Women are the most at risk of being trafficked, coerced into survival sex, and subjected to sexual violence. The fight against trafficking has been underlined as one of the EU's priorities, but large gaps in protection for women victims of trafficking remain. In some cases, for example, accommodation provided for asylum seekers or refugees may not be sufficiently secure and may expose women to risks of sexual assault or violence.[61]

STIs and HIV have become urgent concerns for populations affected by armed conflict and migration because transmission is greater among people in forced migration settings as compared with stable populations.[62] The effects are not limited to refugees themselves, but extend to all those in the conflict or postconflict setting. Poverty, powerlessness, and social instability increase the spread of STIs and HIV. Many governmental bodies recognize the importance of reproductive health services and HIV/AIDS prevention/care services, in particular for refugees; however, in only a few cases have these health policies been translated into practice. Migrants and refugees originating from areas where infections persist can pose a significant challenge for national disease control and elimination strategies.

Female Genital Mutilation/Cutting

Female genital mutilation/cutting (FGM/C) refers to all procedures involving partial or total removal of the external female genitalia for cultural or other nontherapeutic reasons. It has become an issue of increasing concern in host countries because of its harmful consequences on physical, sexual, and psychological health.[63] Many countries that are hosting migrants from places where FGM/C is perpetrated have established guidelines on FGM/C for medical providers. Even though international organizations condemn FGM/C as a violation of human rights, and most nations have banned it, it remains prevalent and is slow to decline in many African countries. This persistence raises questions about the effectiveness of international and national laws prohibiting the practice as well as the potential role of returning migrants in the changing embedded cultural norms.

Migration from countries where FGM/C is practiced to countries where it is not customary or legal, leads to cultural change and declining support of this practice in these groups.[64] In addition, after migration, affected women live in the midst of a dominant discourse categorizing them as "mutilated" and sexually disfigured. Concurrently, there is a strong correlation between a negative body image and sexual dysfunction.[65]

CHRONIC, NONINFECTIOUS DISEASES

The rates of noncommunicable diseases (NCDs) appear to differ between migrants and the host populations in high-income countries. Exposing refugees and migrants to the risks associated with population movements increases their vulnerability to NCDs. Postmigration lifestyle changes in diet and physical activity may influence the risk of NCDs among migrants in a very significant way. Although infectious diseases are the major cause of mortality in sub-Saharan Africa, it is likely that the health transition in migrant populations will see NCDs take over this position.[65,66]

The key issue regarding NCDs in highly mobile populations is the interruption of continuous treatment that is crucial for chronic conditions. Preexisting dermatologic diseases like atopic eczema or psoriasis can become exacerbated because of poor access to health care and medications. Moreover, generalized dermatoses may result in a variety of systemic disorders.[67,68]

Type 2 diabetes is the only disease that is more common in virtually all migrant groups than in the host population. In addition, the age of diabetes onset is 10 to 20 years earlier compared with the host population, and microvascular complications such as peripheral neuropathy and foot ulcers are seen earlier.[67,68]

Some studies report the incidence of infectious disease–related cancers, such as hepatic cancer, Kaposi sarcoma, cervical cancer, and some lymphomas, is higher in migrants than in the host population.[69] This could be attributed to migrants' exposure to infections in early life in their home countries before migration. Skin cancer rates also vary substantially in migrants moving to other latitudes, due to the adoption of risk behaviors of the host country accompanied by lack of knowledge and the belief that dark skin is protective.[70] Prevention, timely detection, and treatment of individuals with NCDs are crucial in improving quality of life and minimizing health care costs associated with NCDs.

SUMMARY

Provision of skin care in migrants and displaced people remains inadequate. Poor access to services and essential medicines, lack of trained health care professionals, linguistic and cultural barriers, human mobility, and legal entitlement to care are the main challenges. Moreover, the process of forced migration exposes refugees and migrants to sexual violence, torture, and exploitation with consequences on skin and sexual health.

The international dermatology community has the duty to raise these issues, prioritize interventions, and increase awareness among stakeholders. With a changing landscape in the climate and demographics, rising political instability and the recent emergence of infectious disease outbreaks, migration will continue to occur. Therefore, advocating for skin health for all and issuing calls for action remain of utmost importance.

DISCLOSURE

The authors declare no commercial or financial conflicts of interest and no funding sources.

REFERENCES

1. UNHCR: Figures at a Glance. Available at: https://www.unhcr.org/en-us/figures-at-a-glance.html. Accessed September 19, 2020.
2. Refugees and Migrants Definitions. Available at: https://refugeesmigrants.un.org/definitions. Accessed September 15, 2019.
3. United Nations Convention and Protocol Relating to the Status of Refugees. 2019. Available at: https://www.unhcr.org/3b66c2aa10. Accessed April 12, 2019.
4. Internally Displaced People. Available at: https://www.unhcr.org/en-us/internally-displaced-people.html. Accessed September 15, 2019.
5. UNHCR: Asylum-Seekers. Available at: https://www.unhcr.org/asylum-seekers.html. Accessed January 31, 2020.
6. UNHCR Refugees and Migrants: Frequently Asked Questions. Available at: https://www.unhcr.org/en-us/news/latest/2016/3/56e95c676/refugees-migrants-frequently-asked-questions-faqs.html. Accessed January 15, 2020.
7. Advancing frontlines, mass exodus and reduced access to hospitals in Idlib. Available at: https://www.msf.org/exodus-and-limited-healthcare-frontline-advances-syria. Accessed February 6, 2020.
8. UNHCR Refugee Facts: Refugee Camps. Available at: https://www.unrefugees.org/refugee-facts/camps/. Accessed January 31, 2020.
9. UNHCR Protracted Refugee Situations Explained. Available at: https://www.unrefugees.org/news/protracted-refugee-situations-explained/. Accessed January 31, 2020.
10. UNHCR Emergency Handbook: Health in Camps. Available at: https://emergency.unhcr.org/entry/54565/health-in-camps. Accessed January 30, 2020.
11. Palazzo Selam: the invisible city. 2014. Available at: https://www.associazionecittadinidelmondo.it/wp-content/uploads/2019/02/Report-Selam-Palace-2014-inglese.pdf. Accessed January 2, 2020.
12. Padovese V, Egidi AM, Melillo Fenech T, et al. Migration and determinants of health: clinical epidemiological characteristics of migrants in Malta (2010-11). J Public Health (Oxf) 2014;36(3):368–74.
13. Di Meco E, Di Napoli A, Amato LM, et al. Infectious and dermatological diseases among arriving migrants on the Italian coasts. Eur J Public Health 2018;28(5):910–6.
14. Kibar Ozturk M. Skin diseases in rural Nyala, Sudan (in a rural hospital, in 12 orphanages, and in two refugee camps). Int J Dermatol 2019;58(11):1341–9.
15. Souliotis K, Saridi M, Banou K, et al. Health and health needs of migrants in detention in Greece: shedding light to an unknown reality. Glob Health 2019;15(1):4.
16. Saikal SL, Ge L, Mir A, et al. Skin disease profile of Syrian refugees in Jordan: a field-mission assessment. J Eur Acad Dermatol Venereol 2020;34(2):419–25.
17. MSF Medical Guidelines, Essential Drugs. Drugs for external use, antiseptics and disinfectants. Available at: https://medicalguidelines.msf.org/viewport/EssDr/english/drugs-for-external-use-antiseptics-and-disinfectants-16688511.html. Accessed January 25, 2020.
18. World Health Organization Model Lists of Essential Medicines. Available at: https://www.who.int/medicines/publications/essentialmedicines/en/. Accessed January 25, 2020.
19. Ternavasio-de-la-Vega HG, Ángel-Moreno A, Hernández-Cabrera M, et al. Skin and soft tissue infections (patera foot) in immigrants, Spain. Emerg Infect Dis 2009;15(4):598–600.
20. Trovato A, Reid A, Takarinda KC, et al. Dangerous crossing: demographic and clinical features of rescued sea migrants seen in 2014 at an outpatient clinic at Augusta Harbor, Italy. Confl Health 2016;10:14.
21. Kousoulis AA, Ioakeim-Ioannidou M, Economopoulos KP. Access to health for refugees in Greece: lessons in inequalities. Int J Equity Health 2016;15(1):122.
22. World Health Organization Child Growth Standards: Methods and development. Available at: https://www.who.int/childgrowth/standards/technical_report/en/. Accessed February 23, 2020.
23. Leidman E, Humphreys A, Greene Cramer B, et al. Acute malnutrition and anemia among Rohingya children in Kutupalong Camp, Bangladesh. JAMA 2018;319(14):1505–6.
24. Weise Prinzo Z, de Benoist B. Meeting the challenges of micronutrient deficiencies in emergency-affected populations. Proc Nutr Soc 2002;61(2):251–7.

25. UNHCR Micronutrient Malnutrition - Detection, Measurement and Intervention. 2003. Available at: https://www.unhcr.org/uk/45fa6dad2.pdf. Accessed February 2, 2020.

26. van den Briel T, Cheung E, Zewari J, et al. Fortifying food in the field to boost nutrition: case studies from Afghanistan, Angola, and Zambia. Food Nutr Bull 2007;28(3):353–64.

27. Seal A, Kafwembe E, Kassim IAR, et al. Maize meal fortification is associated with improved vitamin A and iron status in adolescents and reduced childhood anaemia in a food aid-dependent refugee population. Public Health Nutr 2008;11(7):720–8.

28. Marano N, Angelo K, Merrill RD, et al. Expanding travel medicine in the 21st century to address the health needs of the world's migrants. J Travel Med 2018;25(1).

29. Greenaway C, Castelli F. Infectious diseases at different stages of migration: an expert review. J Trav Med 2019;26(2).

30. Castelli F, Sulis G. Migration and infectious diseases. Clin Microbiol Infect 2017;23(5):283–9.

31. World Health Organization Europe. Migration and health: key issues. Available at: http://www.euro.who.int/en/health-topics/health-determinants/migration-and-health/migrant-health-in-the-european-region/migration-and-health-key-issues. Accessed February 2, 2020.

32. Abbas M, Aloudat T, Bartolomei J, et al. Migrant and refugee populations: a public health and policy perspective on a continuing global crisis. Antimicrob Resist Infect Control 2018;7:113.

33. Norman FF, Comeche B, Chamorro S, et al. Overcoming challenges in the diagnosis and treatment of parasitic infectious diseases in migrants. Expert Rev Anti Infect Ther 2020;18(2):127–43.

34. Zammarchi L, Gobbi F, Angheben A, et al. Schistosomiasis, strongyloidiasis and Chagas disease: the leading imported neglected tropical diseases in Italy. J Travel Med 2020;27(1).

35. Agbata EN, Morton RL, Bisoffi Z, et al. Effectiveness of screening and treatment approaches for schistosomiasis and strongyloidiasis in newly-arrived migrants from endemic countries in the EU/EEA: a systematic review. Int J Environ Res Public Health 2018;16(1).

36. Beeres DT, Ravensbergen SJ, Heidema A, et al. Efficacy of ivermectin mass-drug administration to control scabies in asylum seekers in the Netherlands: A retrospective cohort study between January 2014 - March 2016. PLoS Negl Trop Dis 2018;12(5):e0006401.

37. El Safadi D, Merhabi S, Rafei R, et al. Cutaneous leishmaniasis in north Lebanon: re-emergence of an important neglected tropical disease. Trans R Soc Trop Med Hyg 2019;113(8):471–6.

38. Kanani K, Amr ZS, Shadfan B, et al. Cutaneous leishmaniasis among Syrian refugees in Jordan. Acta Trop 2019;194:169–71.

39. Ozbilgin A, Gencoglan G, Tunali V, et al. Refugees at the crossroads of continents: a molecular approach for cutaneous leishmaniasis among refugees in Turkey. Acta Parasit 2020;65:136–43. https://doi.org/10.2478/s11686-019-00139-4.

40. Lam E, McCarthy A, Brennan M. Vaccine-preventable diseases in humanitarian emergencies among refugee and internally-displaced populations. Hum Vaccin Immunother 2015;11(11):2627–36.

41. Shimakawa Y, Camelique O, Ariyoshi K. Outbreak of chickenpox in a refugee camp of Northern Thailand. Confl Health 2010;4:4.

42. CDC Vaccination Program for U.S.-bound Refugees. Available at: https://www.cdc.gov/immigrantrefugeehealth/guidelines/overseas/interventions/immunizations-schedules.html. Accessed February 1, 2020.

43. Kouadio IK, Kamigaki T, Oshitani H. Measles outbreaks in displaced populations: a review of transmission, morbidity and mortality associated factors. BMC Int Health Hum Rights 2010;10:5.

44. WHO Mortality and Morbidity Weekly Bulletin, Cox's Bazar, Bangladesh. 2017. Available at: http://www.searo.who.int/bangladesh/mmwbvol8.pdf. Accessed January 31, 2020.

45. Chin T, Buckee CO, Mahmud AS. Quantifying the success of measles vaccination campaigns in the Rohingya refugee camps. Epidemics 2020;30:100385.

46. CDC Varicella For HealthCare Professionals. Available at: https://www.cdc.gov/chickenpox/hcp/index.html. Accessed January 25, 2020.

47. CDC Travelers' Health, Travel-Related Infectious Diseases. Varicella (Chickenpox). Available at: https://wwwnc.cdc.gov/travel/yellowbook/2020/travel-related-infectious-diseases/varicella-chickenpox. Accessed January 25, 2020.

48. Cadieux G, Redditt V, Graziano D, et al. Risk factors for varicella susceptibility among refugees to Toronto, Canada. J Immigr Minor Health 2017;19(1):6–14.

49. Hsan K, Naher S, Gozal D, et al. Varicella outbreak among the Rohingya refugees in Bangladesh: lessons learned and potential prevention strategies. Travel Med Infect Dis 2019;31:101465.

50. Lesens O, Baud O, Henquell C, et al. Varicella outbreak in Sudanese refugees from Calais. J Travel Med 2016;23(5).

51. Vairo F, Di Bari V, Panella V, et al. An outbreak of chickenpox in an asylum seeker centre in Italy: outbreak investigation and validity of reported chickenpox history, December 2015-May 2016. Euro Surveill 2017;22(46).

52. de Valliere S, Cani N, Grossenbacher M, et al. Comparison of two strategies to prevent varicella outbreaks in housing facilities for asylum seekers. Int J Infect Dis 2011;15(10):e716–21.

53. Pareek M, Greenaway C, Noori T, et al. The impact of migration on tuberculosis epidemiology and control in high-income countries: a review. BMC Med 2016;14:48.

54. Fakoya I, Álvarez-Del Arco D, Monge S, et al. HIV testing history and access to treatment among migrants living with HIV in Europe. J Int AIDS Soc 2018;21(Suppl 4):e25123.

55. Eiset AH, Wejse C. Review of infectious diseases in refugees and asylum seekers-current status and going forward. Public Health Rev 2017;38:22.

56. Seedat F, Hargreaves S, Nellums LB, et al. How effective are approaches to migrant screening for infectious diseases in Europe? A systematic review. Lancet Infect Dis 2018;18(9):e259–71.

57. Panagiotopoulos T. Screening for infectious diseases in newly arrived migrants in Europe: the context matters. Euro Surveill 2018;23(28).

58. Taylor R, King K, Vodicka P, et al. Screening for leprosy in immigrants–a decision analysis model. Lepr Rev 2003;74(3):240–8.

59. People on the Move: Torture and Migration. Data in the Fight Against Impunity. Available at: https://irct.org/assets/uploads/pdf_20170906095246.pdf. Accessed February 11, 2020.

60. Clarysse K, Grosber M, Ring J, et al. Skin lesions, differential diagnosis and practical approach to potential survivors of torture. J Eur Acad Dermatol Venereol 2019;33(7):1232–40.

61. European Institute for Gender Equality. Gender-specific measures in anti-trafficking actions. Available at: https://ec.europa.eu/anti-trafficking/sites/antitrafficking/files/read_the_report_gender-specific_measures_in_anti-trafficking_actions.pdf. Accessed February 11, 2020.

62. Available at: http://hivinsite.ucsf.edu/InSite-KB-ref.jsp?page=kb-08-01-08&rf=15. Accessed February 22, 2020.

63. World Health Organization. Female genital mutilation. Available at: https://www.who.int/news-room/fact-sheets/detail/female-genital-mutilation. Accessed February 11, 2020.

64. Johansen REB, Ziyada MM, Shell-Duncan B, et al. Health sector involvement in the management of female genital mutilation/cutting in 30 countries. BMC Health Serv Res 2018;18(1):240.

65. Johnsdotter S. The impact of migration on attitudes to female genital cutting and experiences of sexual dysfunction among migrant women with FGC. Curr Sex Health Rep 2018;10(1):18–24.

66. Moullan Y, Jusot F. Why is the 'healthy immigrant effect' different between European countries? Eur J Public Health 2014;24(Suppl 1):80–6.

67. Vandenheede H, Deboosere P, Stirbu I, et al. Migrant mortality from diabetes mellitus across Europe: the importance of socio-economic change. Eur J Epidemiol 2012;27(2):109–17.

68. Agyemang C, van den Born BJ. Non-communicable diseases in migrants: an expert review. J Travel Med 2019;26(2).

69. Kunst AE, Stronks K, Agyemang C. Non-communicable diseases. In: Rechel B, Mladovsky P, Devillé W, et al, editors. Martin McKee.Migration and health in the European Union. Birkshire, England: Open University Press; 2011. p. 101–20.

70. Padovese V, Franco G, Valenzano M, et al. Skin cancer risk assessment in dark skinned immigrants: the role of social determinants and ethnicity. Ethn Health 2018;23(6):649–58.

71. Desenclos JC, Berry AM, Padt R, et al. Epidemiological patterns of scurvy among Ethiopian refugees. Bull World Health Organ 1989;67(3):309–16.

72. Seaman J, Rivers JP. Scurvy and anaemia in refugees. Lancet 1989;1(8648):1204.

73. Seal AJ, Creeke PI, Mirghani Z, et al. Iron and vitamin A deficiency in long-term African refugees. J Nutr 2005;135(4):808–13.

74. Khatib IM, Elmadfa I. High prevalence rates of anemia, vitamin A deficiency and stunting imperil the health status of Bedouin schoolchildren in North Badia, Jordan. Ann Nutr Metab 2009;55(4):358–67.

75. Ververs M, Muriithi JW, Burton A, et al. Scurvy outbreak among South Sudanese adolescents and young men - Kakuma Refugee Camp, Kenya, 2017-2018. MMWR Morb Mortal Wkly Rep 2019;68(3):72–5.

The Impact of Vitiligo on Quality of Life and Psychosocial Well-Being in a Nepalese Population

Jenny Pun, MBBS, MD[a],[*],[1], Aastha Randhawa, MBBS[b],[1], Ajay Kumar, MBBS, MD[a], Victoria Williams, MD[c]

KEYWORDS

- Vitiligo • Psychosocial impact • Awareness • Quality of life • Social discrimination • Marriage

KEY POINTS

- In a Nepalese cohort, vitiligo patients were predominantly young adult men from urban or semiurban areas with high school or above education.
- The Vitiligo Quality of Life (VitiQoL) and Vitiligo Impact Scale (VIS) instruments did not reveal an overall large impact of vitiligo on quality of life for the participants.
- Focused surveys, however, revealed most patients felt worried or unhappy, experienced social stigma, faced difficulty in gaining employment and finding a life partner, believed myths or superstitions about vitiligo, and had inadequate counseling by their health care providers.
- Information gathered through semistructured interviews centered around the major theme of psychosocial distress experienced by patients due to social discrimination and stigmatization, misinformation on vitiligo, and untreated mental health concerns.

INTRODUCTION

Vitiligo is a relatively common acquired disorder of pigmentation characterized by the development of well-defined depigmented macules and patches on the skin. Lesions may occur in a localized or generalized distribution and may coalesce into large, depigmented areas. In Nepal, information on vitiligo is limited and there exists no formal epidemiologic data on the prevalence and incidence. One study reported the overall prevalence of skin diseases in rural Nepal was 20.1% and pigmentary disorders, such as vitiligo, were among the top 10 most common skin diseases.[1] Kumar and colleagues[2] found that generalized vitiligo is the most common clinical subtype found in western Nepal.

Patients with a visible chronic skin disease often experience discrimination and stigmatization resulting in psychosocial impairments in addition to their physical burden of disease.[3,4] The highly visible nature of vitiligo allows for significant psychosocial impact, particularly in a country like Nepal, where it is the authors' experience that society generally stereotypes physical appearances across all aspects of life. In the neighboring country of India, which shares a common socioeconomic and cultural background with Nepal, studies have shown that vitiligo patients commonly experience psychiatric morbidity, including depression, embarrassment, social problems, cognitive impairment, physical limitation, discomfort, anger, and fear.[5] It is the authors'

[a] Department of Dermatology, Manipal Teaching Hospital, Fulbari, Pokhara-11, Kaski 33700, Nepal; [b] Department of Dermatology, Manipal College of Medical Sciences, Manipal Teaching Hospital, Fulbari, Pokhara-11, Kaski 33700, Nepal; [c] Department of Dermatology, Perelman School of Medicine at the University of Pennsylvania, 2 Maloney Building, 3600 Spruce St, Philadelphia, PA 19104, USA
[1] These authors contributed equally.
* Corresponding author.
E-mail address: jenniferderma98@gmail.com

Dermatol Clin 39 (2021) 117–127
https://doi.org/10.1016/j.det.2020.08.011

experience that patients with vitiligo in Nepal are faced with similar stigma, leading to embarrassment, self-consciousness, anxiety, and depression. One study found that more than half of patients reported serious economic and financial consequences due to their vitiligo. These effects were more common in women and those with generalized disease.[5]

Lack of awareness and understanding of vitiligo also is a problem for Nepalese patients. Agrawal and colleagues[6] concluded that more than 60% of patients with vitiligo in Nepal believed that their skin disease was caused by "germs or virus," whereas 50% of them thought that it was due to "chance or fate." It is the authors' belief that myths and misunderstandings about vitiligo can have detrimental effects on quality of life; however, the extent of this has not been fully explored in Nepal.

The authors' study aims to fill a gap in knowledge on the epidemiologic patterns of vitiligo and the psychosocial impact of this disease on a cohort of patients with vitiligo in midwestern Nepal. The specific objectives of the study include (1) describing the baseline demographics of the vitiligo cohort, (2) quantitatively measuring the psychosocial impact of vitiligo on the cohort, (3) qualitatively describing the major psychosocial concerns that arise due to vitiligo in the cohort, and, most importantly, (4) describing how this campaign was designed and implemented to educate the patient population about their skin disease and spread awareness of vitiligo to the general public.

METHODS
Study Design

The authors used a cross-sectional survey design to describe the demographics and clinical features and measure the psychosocial impact of vitiligo in the cohort. They used qualitative semistructured interviews to describe the psychosocial concerns that arise due to vitiligo in a cohort.

Study Setting and Participants

The study was conducted at Manipal Teaching Hospital located in Pokhara, a moderate sized urban area in midwestern Nepal. The authors used an annual Vitiligo Awareness campaign as a platform to invite patients with a diagnosis of vitiligo to participate in the study, consisting of a questionnaire on demographic/clinical data, the Vitiligo Impact Scale (VIS) and Vitiligo Quality of Life (VitiQoL) index surveys.[7,8] Participants additionally were invited to participate in a 1-on-1 semistructured interview. The entire session concluded with educational didactics. Patients who did not

have a diagnosis of vitiligo, were not participating in the Vitiligo Awareness campaign, had a preexisting psychiatric morbidity that did not stem from skin pathology, and did not consent to share information were excluded from the study.

Data Collection

A focused survey created by study investigators collected the following data variables: age, gender, marital status, education, age of onset, place of residence, any previous medical or psychiatric illness, and medication history. The authors also surveyed participants about their beliefs on the causation/spread of vitiligo, their life challenges faced, and experience with previous medical treatments. Two quantitative survey instruments were used as tools to measure the psychosocial impact of vitiligo: the VitiQoL and VIS. The VIS is an instrument used to assess the psychosocial burden of vitiligo, whereas the VitiQoL is a vitiligo-specific quality-of-life instrument.[7,8] The VitiQoL scale has been validated on large samples of patients both in the United States and internationally and consists of 15 questions with a 7-point Likert scale (0–6). The scores range from 0 to 90; higher scores represent poorer quality of life. The VIS was developed and validated in the Indian population and has shown similar internal consistency for its items as the VitiQoL scale. The VIS has 27 items, with each item scored from 0 to 3; scores range from 0 to 81, with higher scores indicating higher psychosocial impact. All patients who were enrolled agreed to fill out surveys and undergo interviews. After obtaining informed consent, participants were interviewed in a private 1-on-1 setting. Open-ended leads were used, as listed in **Fig. 1**, to probe their level of insight, baseline awareness, and understanding of the etiology and prognosis of vitiligo. The participants were encouraged to share their feelings and emotions in relation to the impact of the disease on their lives. Interview notes were recorded on paper by medical student volunteers and transcribed thereafter for thematic analysis by study investigators.

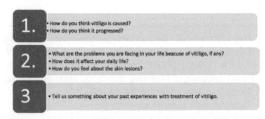

1.
• How do you think vitiligo is caused?
• How do you think it progressed?

2.
• What are the problems you are facing in your life beacuse of vitiligo, if any?
• How does it affect your daily life?
• How do you feel about the skin lesions?

3
• Tell us something about your past experiences with treatment of vitiligo.

Fig. 1. Overview of the main open-ended interview questions.

Data Analysis

Demographic data was reported using means and standard deviations (SDs) for continuous variables or percentages for counts. Age and gender have previously been shown to have a significant impact on quality of life in people suffering from vitiligo.[9,10] Multivariate linear regression models, therefore, were created to study the relationship between quantitative scores of vitiligo quality of life, accounting for the potential confounding effects of age and gender. Gender differences in VIS and VitiQoL also were assessed separately with Student *t* tests. The authors studied the correlation of educational status with both VIS and VitiQoL, owing to previous studies, indicating strong associations between low educational status and depression.[11] Statistical analyses were performed using R version 3.6 statistical software.[12] Qualitative data were analyzed using the principles of thematic analysis of Braun and Clarke[13] to define shared thematic elements across their narratives. Final themes where identified after iterative steps involving transcription of data, coding and data reduction, generation of initial themes, and review and of the themes in context of the total data set.

Ethical Considerations

Ethics approval was obtained from the Manipal institutional review board. Written consent was obtained from all participants prior to study participation.

THE VITILIGO AWARENESS CAMPAIGN

The campaign consisted of 2 events held on World Vitiligo Day, the 25th of June of 2018 and of 2019 (**Fig. 2**). Both were designed to have segments in which the participants speak about their intrapersonal and social problems. The authors wanted them to freely communicate and report their day-to-day issues relevant to the disease. The first event, held in 2018, was aimed to be easy to accomplish, meaningful, and impactful. The event included educational discussions, medical student participation, support material (**Fig. 3**), and incentives, such as a photobooth (**Fig. 4**), campaign T-shirts, and cosmetic gift bags for the patients. The second campaign was designed to target the issues brought up by patients during the initial campaign in a more systematic way, including those discussed in the following sections with data collection for this study.

Clinical Care and Education

Clinical care and educatoin included an educational briefing on vitiligo: causes, risk factors, prognosis, and treatments options for vitiligo. A full medical examination along with a panel of laboratory tests, such as complete blood cell count and thyroid function test, were conducted in order to diagnose other potentially associated autoimmune diseases and comorbidities (data from these tests are not included in this study). Clinicians used focused surveys to record demographic and vitiligo-related psychosocial factors during examinations.

Psychiatric Evaluation and Breakout Session

The patients were given motivational speeches and the psychosocial impact of vitiligo was evaluated through the VIS and VitiQoL surveys. Participant interviews were conducted 1-on-1 to discuss concerns related to the disease, as described previously. People who expressed a desire for mental health support were additionally provided professional counseling.

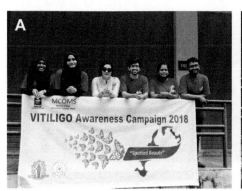
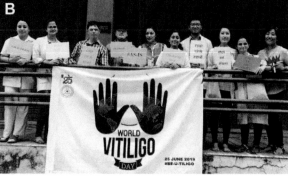

Fig. 2. (*A*) The organizing faculty member, Dr Jenny Pun, along with student volunteers welcoming participants to the first vitiligo awareness campaign in Pokhara, Nepal. (*B*) Vitiligo patients along with faculty, residents, and nurses after the second vitiligo awareness campaign, held in 2019.

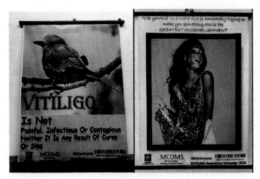

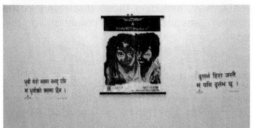

Fig. 3. Simple illustrative posters displayed at the hallway for spreading vitiligo awareness among the general public and passing by.

Reflective Peer Support Group Session

The reflective peer support group sessions were oriented toward participants' external struggles (families, community, and professional interactions) with an aim of helping them deal with the social barriers surrounding their stigmatized disease. For many, this was their first chance to vocalize their struggles and served as a therapeutic form of self-expression and self-empowerment.

RESULTS
Demographics

Of 22 patients who enrolled in the study during the campaign, 59.1% (13/22) were male, with a mean age of 38.7 years (SD 3.2). The mean age of onset of vitiligo skin lesions was 26.2 years (SD 3.2). A majority had completed high school education (77.3%; 17/22) and many were married (68.2%; 15/22). Approximately 17 out of 22 (77.3%) of the participants were residents of Pokhara or regions within 10 km of the city center, whereas only a few came from outside of the area. All 22 participants completed the surveys and interviews. Full demographic details are summarized in **Table 1**.

Psychosocial Features

Table 2 presents psychosocial concerns and health behaviors of participants related to vitiligo. All participants reported facing some form of social discrimination or stigmatization by others (100%; 22/22), and 9% (2/22) were ill-treated even by their immediate family. Multiple concurrent misunderstandings about the etiology/contagion of vitiligo were common, including beliefs that it is caused by supernatural forces (68.2%;15/22), diet (63.6%; 14/22), and related to leprosy (22.7%; 5/22). There also was fear or guilt about the potential to spread vitiligo through physical contact (13.6%; 3/22). Participants commonly reported negative thoughts and emotions, including low self-esteem (72.7%; 16/22) and worry/unhappiness related to their skin condition (68.2%; 15/22). Major concerns included difficulties in finding a partner (81.8%; 18/22) and obtaining employment (54.5%; 12/22). Twelve out of 22 participants (54.5%) had changed more than 2 doctors as they were unsatisfied with their treatment, and 16 out of 22 (71.7%) felt that they were not counseled properly by their treating doctor. Some patients had discontinued treatment because they were unable to bear the cost of medications (36.3%; 8/22).

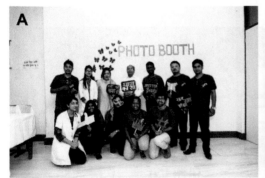

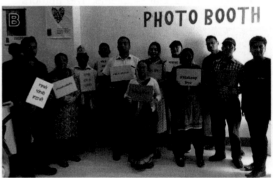

Fig. 4. (*A*) Members of the Department of Dermatology at Manipal Teaching Hospital posing along with medical students at the photobooth, which was used to engage vitiligo participants in the 2018 Vitiligo Awareness campaign. (*B*) Members of the Department of Psychiatry at Manipal Teaching Hospital with vitiligo patients at the photobooth, made for the 2019 Vitiligo Awareness campaign. Residents of the psychiatry department were invited to provide psychological counseling, under the guidance of faculty members.

Table 1
Demographic details of participants with vitiligo in Nepal

Category	Variables	N (%); *Total N = 22*
Participant age (Mean +/- SD, y)	38.7 ± 3.2	
Age of onset (Mean +/- SD, y)	26.2 ± 3.2	
Marital status	Married	15 (68.2)
	Unmarried	6 (27.3)
	Divorced	1 (4.5)
Sex	Male	13 (59.1)
	Female	9 (40.1)
Education level	None	2 (9.1)
	Up to high school	17 (77.3)
	Graduated	1 (4.5)
	Postgraduate	2 (9.1)
Residence location (in reference to Pokhara)	Within 10 km	17 (77.3)
	Outside 10 km but within the district	3 (13.6)
	Outside of the district	2 (9.1)

Participants had a mean VitiQoL score of 37.2 ± 24.2 and mean VIS scores of 23.9 ± 15.9, which both correspond to a lower-level impact on quality of life. **Fig. 5** summarizes the distribution of responses for individual questions of the VitiQoL and VIS surveys. Individual questions with the highest (most impactful) scores on the VitiQoL survey were question 15, indicating that 68.2% of participants were worried about the progression of their disease, and question 8, indicating that 40.9% felt vitiligo affected their choice of clothing. High-impact

Table 2
Survey responses reflecting psychosocial concerns and health behaviors of participants with vitiligo in Nepal

Vitiligo Question Categories	Specific Responses	N (%); *Total N = 22*
Beliefs/concerns about causation and spread	God/supernatural involvement	15 (68.2)
	Dietary involvement	14 (63.6)
	Relation to leprosy	5 (22.7)
	Genetic cause	18 (81.8)
	Fear or guilt of spreading through physical contact	3 (13.6)
Life challenges faced	Social discrimination and stigmatization	22 (100)
	Difficulty getting married/ finding a partner	18 (81.8)
	Discrimination within immediate family	2 (9.1)
	Difficulty getting jobs	12 (54.5)
	Low self-esteem	16 (72.7)
	Feeling unhappy or worried	15 (68.2)
Previous experience with medical treatment	Satisfied with treatment	10 (45.4)
	Changed doctors more than 2 times	12 (54.5)
	Inadequate counseling by the health care provider	16 (71.7)
	Noncompliance due to cost of treatment	8 (36.3)

A

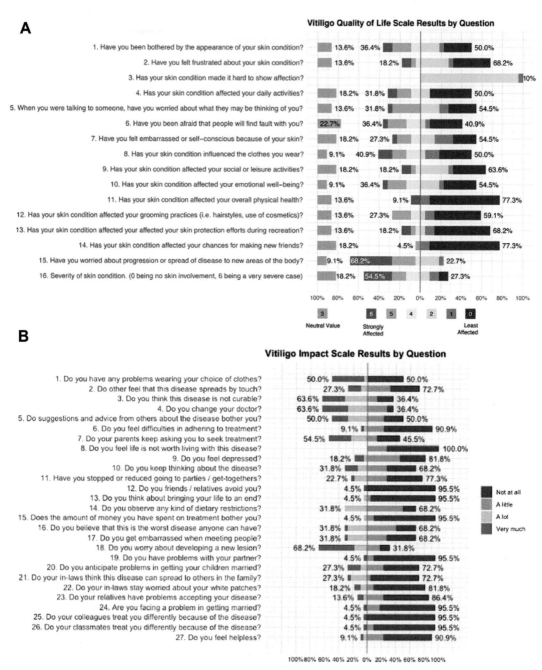

Vitiligo Quality of Life Scale Results by Question

1. Have you been bothered by the appearance of your skin condition? 13.6% 36.4% 50.0%
2. Have you felt frustrated about your skin condition? 13.6% 18.2% 68.2%
3. Has your skin condition made it hard to show affection? 10%
4. Has your skin condition affected your daily activities? 18.2% 31.8% 50.0%
5. When you were talking to someone, have you worried about what they may be thinking of you? 13.6% 31.8% 54.5%
6. Have you been afraid that people will find fault with you? 22.7% 36.4% 40.9%
7. Have you felt embarrassed or self–conscious because of your skin? 18.2% 27.3% 54.5%
8. Has your skin condition influenced the clothes you wear? 9.1% 40.9% 50.0%
9. Has your skin condition affected your social or leisure activities? 18.2% 18.2% 63.6%
10. Has your skin condition affected your emotional well–being? 9.1% 36.4% 54.5%
11. Has your skin condition affected your overall physical health? 13.6% 9.1% 77.3%
12. Has your skin condition affected your grooming practices (i.e. hairstyles, use of cosmetics)? 13.6% 27.3% 59.1%
13. Has your skin condition affected your affected your skin protection efforts during recreation? 13.6% 18.2% 68.2%
14. Has your skin condition affected your chances for making new friends? 18.2% 4.5% 77.3%
15. Have you worried about progression or spread of disease to new areas of the body? 9.1% 68.2% 22.7%
16. Severity of skin condition. (0 being no skin involvement, 6 being a very severe case) 18.2% 54.5% 27.3%

100% 80% 60% 40% 20% 0% 20% 40% 60% 80% 100%

| 3 | | 6 | 5 | 4 | 2 | 1 | 0 |

Neutral Value   Strongly Affected   Least Affected

B

Vitiligo Impact Scale Results by Question

1. Do you have any problems wearing your choice of clothes? 50.0% 50.0%
2. Do other feel that this disease spreads by touch? 27.3% 72.7%
3. Do you think this disease is not curable? 63.6% 36.4%
4. Do you change your doctor? 63.6% 36.4%
5. Do suggestions and advice from others about the disease bother you? 50.0% 50.0%
6. Do you feel difficulties in adhering to treatment? 9.1% 90.9%
7. Do your parents keep asking you to seek treatment? 54.5% 45.5%
8. Do you feel life is not worth living with this disease? 100.0%
9. Do you feel depressed? 18.2% 81.8%
10. Do you keep thinking about the disease? 31.8% 68.2%
11. Have you stopped or reduced going to parties / get-togethers? 22.7% 77.3%
12. Do your friends / relatives avoid you? 4.5% 95.5%
13. Do you think about bringing your life to an end? 4.5% 95.5%
14. Do you observe any kind of dietary restrictions? 31.8% 68.2%
15. Does the amount of money you have spent on treatment bother you? 4.5% 95.5%
16. Do you believe that this is the worst disease anyone can have? 31.8% 68.2%
17. Do you get embarrassed when meeting people? 31.8% 68.2%
18. Do you worry about developing a new lesion? 68.2% 31.8%
19. Do you have problems with your partner? 4.5% 95.5%
20. Do you anticipate problems in getting your children married? 27.3% 72.7%
21. Do your in-laws think this disease can spread to others in the family? 27.3% 72.7%
22. Do your in-laws stay worried about your white patches? 18.2% 81.8%
23. Do your relatives have problems accepting your disease? 13.6% 86.4%
24. Are you facing a problem in getting married? 4.5% 95.5%
25. Do your colleagues treat you differently because of the disease? 4.5% 95.5%
26. Do your classmates treat you differently because of the disease? 4.5% 95.5%
27. Do you feel helpless? 9.1% 90.9%

Not at all
A little
A lot
Very much

100% 80% 60% 40% 20% 0% 20% 40% 60% 80% 100%

Fig. 5. (*A*) VitiQoL score breakdown by question, illustrating greater impact on quality of life with a greater proportional left shift in blue. (*B*) VIS score breakdown by question, illustrating greater impact on quality of life with a greater proportional left shift in blue.

scores on the VIS survey were question 18, in which 68.2% of participants indicated a fear of developing new lesions; question 3, where 63.6% believed that vitiligo is incurable; and question 4, which indicated that 63.6% changed doctors frequently. The relationship between Viti-QoL scores and age, and VIS scores and age were analyzed using 2 linear regression models, with gender as an additional covariate. The relationship of both VitiQoL and VIS with age was nonsignificant (adjusted R^2 = 0.10 and P value = .48, and adjusted R^2 = 0.08 and P value = .11, respectively). Gender differences in scores on the VIS and VitiQoL also were found to be nonsignificant using Student *t* tests (P = .28 and P = .061, respectively). Finally, the relationship of educational qualifications with the VIS and VitiQoL scores also were found to be nonsignificant respectively.

THEMES FROM PATIENT NARRATIVES

An overall theme of psychological distress was uncovered in participant interviews with subthemes centered around the impact of stigma/discrimination and misunderstandings about vitiligo (summarized in **Fig. 6**).

The Impact of Stigma and Discrimination

Men and loss of the army dream
In Nepal, many young men aspire to be accepted as a member of the armed forces because it is regarded as a badge of honor and prestige within Nepalese communities. Additionally, the army often is the only way young men escape the village life and move up the socioeconomic ladder. In Nepal, discriminatory regulations persist that prevent people with visible skin disorders from qualifying to join the Nepalese army. The authors found that participants felt discouraged and helpless that features of their physical appearance were being viewed as a disability preventing them from joining the army. This in turn contributed to lower self-esteem: "I am 35 years and I spent my teenage years preparing to get into the Army. I was around 20 when I developed vitiligo starting from my lower limbs, only to find out that I could not apply for the Army anymore. I saw a newspaper article also, stating that people with vitiligo cannot apply for the Army. I fail to understand why they wouldn't want an otherwise fit and healthy person, who is willing to serve his nation."

Women and marriage difficulty
In Nepal, marriage is a major life goal, particularly for young women who often see it as a path to a higher social status and necessary to attain respect from their family/community. The female participants reported more emotional distress around the topic of marriage compared with male participants. Most female participants were unmarried or divorced and strongly felt that vitiligo was the cause. One woman reported being recently divorced right after her diagnosis. Another middle-aged woman, burst into tears while she recounted her experiences: "I got married at 15 years of age according to the customs of my local community, and while it was all going well, I started to develop symptoms of vitiligo. I was tortured in my husband's house as they thought it was communicable and I have brought bad luck to the house. Eventually I was given a divorce at the age of 16 years and I could not remarry ever because of the stigmatization."

Vitiligo and Untreated Mental Health Concerns

Approximately 75% of vitiligo patients are known to have psychological disorders, and studies have shown that counseling can help improve body image, self-esteem, and the quality of life of patients with vitiligo.[14] The participants reported signs/symptoms of low self-esteem and depressive moods, which were concerning for undiagnosed depression. Almost none had previously disclosed that they had a mental health concern or sought counseling. One middle-aged woman appeared quite upset about her disease but did not want to overtly acknowledge it: "I do not feel like doing anything, I don't want to visit the public places much or go to public events. I feel myself zoning out and being inattentive to the events around me. Though my family is supportive of my disease, I keep thinking about the times I did not have this."

The Impact of Misinformation About Vitiligo

Myths about causation
A majority of participants held some inaccurate beliefs in myths about the cause of vitiligo. The most common recurring themes observed were vitiligo being a "curse of God," having dietary association especially with fish and milk, and being related to leprosy. These erroneous beliefs contributed to low self-esteem and psychological distress. A 72-year-old man was brought to the campaign by his daughter-in-law who told the authors that, "He believes it to be a curse of his ancestors and a consequence of him selling their land."

Beliefs about treatment
In the campaign, a majority of patients expressed an awareness that vitiligo was not curable;

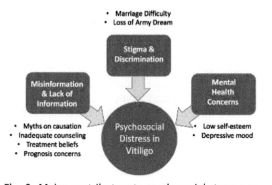

Fig. 6. Major contributors to psychosocial stress associated with vitiligo in a Nepalese population.

however, many still sought out multiple doctors and had tried various traditional medicine treatments, such as Ayurvedic medicine, homeopathic medicine, and Buddhist healing practices. Patients reported that despite understanding their prognosis, they did not want to give up hope that a treatment could one day cure them. For those who used allopathic medicines, there was significant dissatisfaction due to a perceived lack of efficacy and the high cost of medications.

Inadequate counseling

Most patients expressed that communication and counseling from their health care providers was lacking. As reported by a woman in her mid-40s, "The doctor I went to scribbled down names of two medicines on the prescription sheet. I am not sure what to expect out of this treatment, but the OPD [outpatient department] was busy and time was short." Participants reported that traditional healers spent much more time with them discussing their condition compared to medical doctors and commonly offered a false sense of hope for a cure. When medical doctors failed to provide them with a strong understanding of their disease, patients felt that they were more likely to fall prey to expensive and ineffective treatments from traditional healers.

Concerns about prognosis

The interviews also revealed differing concerns regarding the implications of being diagnosed with an incurable skin disease. Younger patients were more concerned about the effects it could have on their appearance and career. In contrast, older patients were more focused on stigma from society and a fear of spreading the disease to their families, as illustrated by a 68-year-old grandfather, who reported, "I make sure I don't kiss my grandchildren, don't want to risk spreading it to them."

DISCUSSION

The authors' study revealed that this Nepalese patient cohort was predominantly young adults who developed vitiligo in their late 20s, an observation in line with a recent Indian study about epidemiologic patterns of vitiligo. That study, however, also showed a female majority, unlike the authors' study, where there was a predominance of male participants.[15] Most of the authors' participants were from within 10 km of the city, which covers a very small percentage of Nepal's terrain, which has many inaccessible rural mountainous regions. This urban bias is reflective of the fact that access to health care and the vitiligo support campaign

was significantly easier for participants in these more urban compared with rural areas of Nepal.[16] In stark contrast to the prevailing literacy rates in the midwestern region of Nepal, a majority of the patients had at least attended high school, and some graduated with degrees, skewing the study toward the educated.[17] Although a majority (68.2%) were married, the divorce rate of 4.5% in the vitiligo cohort was significant compared with the national divorce rate of 0.1% in Nepal. This is consistent with the interview theme of vitiligo and marriage, which focused on women fearing that their skin disease would damage their marriage, especially women who were discriminated against by their spouses and in-laws, hence, highlighting the negative psychosocial impact of vitiligo on relationships.[18]

Previous research in societies with similar socioeconomic compositions have established that vitiligo can lead to psychosocial distress, including social anxiety, feelings of rejection/ isolation, and depression.[19,20] Overall, the authors' results are consistent with these findings. Through a combination of interviews and surveys, the participants indicated psychosocial distress centered around subthemes of social stigma/discrimination, untreated mental health concerns, and misinformation about vitiligo. The authors found that these stressors were present both at the individual level (low self-esteem, interpersonal relationship problems, and employment) and on a larger social scale (stigma, discrimination, misinformation, and myths). Specific concerns focused heavily around the social effects of stigma, including difficulty getting a job, difficulty securing a life partner, loss of social status, and fears of others not wanting to have physical contact with them. These features indicate that patient concerns have a predominantly external social focus, reflective of the authors' experiences of Nepalese culture, which is highly concerned with perceived image. The signs of low-self-esteem and depressive moods in the participants raised concerns for untreated mental health disorders. The uncertainty of vitiligo's disease course has been reported as a major contributor to negative emotions and this was reflected by the misinformation about etiology/prognosis/treatment of vitiligo that the participants experienced.[21,22] Concerningly, a study from India demonstrated that the mood problems and poor coping mechanisms of vitiligo patients can even result in suicidal ideation.[19] Thus, the authors have identified increasing access to mental health counseling as an area of possible intervention that could improve quality of life in the cohort.

Interviews and surveys indicated that the patients had significant misconceptions regarding the etiology and spread of vitiligo. Many participants believed that they developed vitiligo due to something that they did wrong, like their diet, or being "cursed" by supernatural power. Perhaps most devastating to those affected is the perceived association with leprosy infection, which is one of the most stigmatized diseases in Nepal.[23] A study done in Saudi Arabia showed similar misconceptions of vitiligo being infectious and having dietary involvement.[24] This is in contrast to work from Iran, where patients believed that stress and genetic background were the main factors responsible for their disease.[12] The authors' study reveals that there is not much improvement in knowledge about vitiligo in the Nepalese population compared with a study conducted in 2016, which showed high rates of similar misconceptions about the etiology and prognosis.[6]

The authors found major indicators of psychosocial distress during interviews and focused surveys, but the objective measures of significant overall quality-of-life disturbances related to vitiligo were lacking. The VIS (23.9 ± 15.9) and VitiQoL scores (37.2 ± 24.2) were relatively low. These low scores are in line with the VIS and VitiQoL scores reported by other cohorts within the Indian subcontinent.[7] In contrast, South American cohorts displayed higher VitiQoL scores (mean VitiQoL of 40.04 ± 27.32), indicating more quality-of-life disturbances related to vitiligo may be present in these regions.[25,26] Although the overall objective survey measures did not indicate a significant negative quality-of-life impact, when scores were broken down, important trends were observed. For both the VitiQoL and VIS, questions rated highest (most impactful) indicated concern and distress surrounding society's perceptions, stigma about the patient's visible skin disease, and inadequate counseling provided by the treating physicians, which correlate well with major themes uncovered during interviews. The differing results on the overall VIS and VitiQoL scores also could be related to patients feeling hesitant or having difficulty quantifying their feelings through numbered scales on the objective surveys and feeling more comfortable to freely express their psychosocial concerns in a responsive discourse during interviews.

A major contribution of the campaign was the opportunity for participants to fill knowledge gaps about their skin disease and openly express previously unaddressed issues, such as social stigmatization. The response was overwhelmingly positive. Over the course of the 2 campaigns, the authors observed that patients appeared to become more comfortable in their skin and more open to expressing their feelings and participating in educative sessions (**Fig. 7**). This campaign also grabbed the attention of the national media. It was promoted by social media role models and influencers within the country, which have a great ability to reach the masses to increase vitiligo awareness and promote destigmatization and social inclusion. After the first campaign, there were more events and media coverage the following year. As a direct result of the publicity garnered, there subsequently was a significant increase in the inflow of patients to the dermatology clinics.

This campaign and the results of the authors' study have fueled the creation of new objectives toward improving quality of life of vitiligo patients in Nepal so that they can live confident, healthy, and productive lives:

- To create more awareness campaigns in remote areas
- To train more volunteers as educated manpower to spread the awareness campaign objectives in their local communities
- To encourage government and nongovernment organization funding to promote the cause at a larger scale

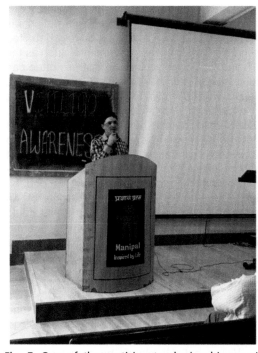

Fig. 7. One of the participants, sharing his experiences about vitiligo and expressing his opinion regarding the need of awareness about this disease.

- To encourage the government to revise and revisit the policies regarding skin diseases
- To improve methods of identification of vitiligo patients with psychosocial distress and refer for appropriate counseling
- To develop events that will help to eradicate social stigma by tackling the cultural myths and misperceptions on vitiligo in local society

LIMITATIONS

Limitations of the study include its small sample size, leading to difficulty generalizing the conclusions to other populations, and a low power to detect relationships between VitiQoL or VIS and age/gender. Further studies on a larger sample of patients across Nepal are needed to fully investigate quality of life in vitiligo.

SUMMARY AND IMPLICATIONS

The authors' cohort of vitiligo patients predominantly were young adult men with some education who experienced psychosocial distress and faced many day-to-day problems as a consequence of their visible skin disease. The most important contributors to psychosocial distress were social discrimination and stigmatization, misinformation on vitiligo, and untreated mental health concerns, summarized in **Fig. 6**. The importance of recognizing this psychosocial distress through open dialogues with patients is highlighted, because it may not be fully detected with quantitative survey instruments, such as the VIS and VitiQoL Psychosocial distress often can go undiagnosed in developing countries like Nepal, which have limited health care resources to allocate to dermatology and mental health. To best of the authors' knowledge, this is the first study of its kind in Nepal to combine a vitiligo awareness campaign and educational event with meaningful data collection to further knowledge about this prevalent disease in the population. The authors present the design of an awareness campaign as an example that could be a model for others looking to increase education and awareness for visible skin diseases like vitiligo in their patient populations.

CLINICS CARE POINTS

- Vitiligo patients should be counselled and screened for clinically significant psychological distress.
- Vitiligo patients should be provided with in depth information about their disease pathogenesis and prognosis, so they can formulate

realistic expectations for their long-term prognosis and treatment outcomes.

- Clinicians should attempt to educate families to prevent isolation and discrimination against patients with vitiligo.

DISCLOSURE

The authors have nothing to disclose.

REFERENCES

1. P Shrestha PD, Mahesh Maskey AK. Skin Diseases: Prevalence and Impact in the Quality of Life of the Community Members in a Rural VDC Final Report.; 2009. https://doi.org/10.1007/s00132-009-1493-8.
2. Kumar A, Neupane S, Parajuli S, et al. Profile of vitiligo in Western Nepal. Nepal J Dermatology, Venereol Leprol 1970;9(1):40–3.
3. Dahlin ME, Runeson B, Firth-Cozens J, et al. Burnout and psychiatric morbidity among medical students entering clinical training: a three year prospective questionnaire and interview-based study. BMC Med Educ 2007;7(1):6.
4. Quality of life in patients with vitiligo: an analysis of the dermatology life quality index outcome over the past two decades. 2016;55(6).
5. Sarkar S, Sarkar T, Sarkar A, et al. Vitiligo and Psychiatric Morbidity: A Profile from a Vitiligo Clinic of a Rural-based Tertiary Care Center of Eastern India. Indian J Dermatol 2018;63(4):281–4. https://doi.org/10.4103/ijd.IJD_142_18.
6. Agrawal S, Kumar A, Shyngwa P. Understanding of nepalese patients with vitiligo about their disease. Nepal J Dermatology, Venereol Leprol 2016;12(1):7–13.
7. Krishna GS, Ramam M, Mehta M, et al. Vitiligo impact scale: An instrument to assess the psychosocial burden of vitiligo. Indian J Dermatol Venereol Leprol 2013;79(2):205–10.
8. Lilly E, Lu PD, Borovicka JH, et al. Development and validation of a vitiligo-specific quality-of-life instrument (VitiQoL). J Am Acad Dermatol 2013;69(1):e11–8. https://doi.org/10.1016/j.jaad.2012.01.038.
9. Sawant NS, Vanjari NA, Khopkar U. Gender differences in depression, coping, stigma, and quality of life in patients of vitiligo. Dermatol Res Pract 2019;2019. https://doi.org/10.1155/2019/6879412.
10. Parsad D, Pandhi R, Dogra S, et al. Dermatology Life Quality Index score in vitiligo and its impact on the treatment outcome [9]. Br J Dermatol 2003;148(2):373–4.
11. Bjelland I, Krokstad S, Mykletun A, et al. Does a higher educational level protect against anxiety and depression? The HUNT study. Soc Sci Med 2008;66(6):1334–45.

12. R Core Team, 2016. R: A Language and Environment for Statistical Computing, Vienna, Austria. Available at: https://www.R-project.org/.

13. Braun V, Clarke V. Using thematic analysis in psychology. Qual Res Psychol 2006;3(2):77–101.

14. Barankin B, DeKoven J. Psychosocial effect of common skin diseases. Can Fam Physician 2002;48:712–6.

15. Kumar S, Nayak C, Padhi T, et al. Epidemiological pattern of psoriasis, vitiligo and atopic dermatitis in India: Hospital-based point prevalence. Indian Dermatol Online J 2014;5(5):6.

16. Bentley H. The organisation of health care in Nepal. Int J Nurs Stud 1995;32(3):260–70.

17. Dhakal B. Statistical trends in literacy rates in Nepal. J Appl Chem 2018;11(11):71–7.

18. Issn O. Interface - Comunicação , Saúde , Educação Vitiligo as a psychosocial disease : apprehensions of patients imprinted by the white O vitiligo como uma doença psicossocial : apreensões de. 2019.

19. Pahwa P, Mehta M, Khaitan BK, et al. The psychosocial impact of vitiligo in Indian patients. Indian J Dermatol Venereol Leprol 2013;79(5):679–85.

20. Journal I, Practice N. Investigating factors associated with quality of life of vitiligo About Wiley Online Library Help & Support. Int J Nurs Pract. 19(S3):3-10.

21. Salman A, Kurt E, Topcuoglu V, et al. Social anxiety and quality of life in vitiligo and acne patients with facial involvement: a cross-sectional controlled study. Am J Clin Dermatol 2016;17(3):305–11.

22. Thompson AR, Clarke SA, Newell RJ, et al. Vitiligo linked to stigmatization in British South Asian women: A qualitative study of the experiences of living with vitiligo. Br J Dermatol 2010;163(3):481–6.

23. Adhikari B, Kaehler N, Chapman RS, et al. Factors affecting perceived stigma in leprosy affected persons in Western Nepal. PLoS Negl Trop Dis 2014;8(6):2–9.

24. Fatani MI, Aldhahri RM, Al Otaibi HO, et al. Acknowledging popular misconceptions about vitiligo in western Saudi Arabia. J Dermatol Surg 2016;20(1):27–31.

25. Gupta V, Sreenivas V, Mehta M, et al. What do Vitiligo Impact Scale-22 scores mean? Studying the clinical interpretation of scores using an anchor-based approach. Br J Dermatol 2019;180(3):580–5.

26. Boza JC, Fabbrin A, Giongo N, et al. Translation, cross-cultural adaptation and validation of the vitiligo-specifi c health-related quality of life instrument (Vitiqol) into brazilian portuguese. An Bras Dermatol 2015;90(3):358–62.

Factors Affecting Quality of Life for People Living with Albinism in Botswana

Ellen E. Anshelevich, BA[a], Karen I. Mosojane, MBBS[b],
Lorato Kenosi, MSocSci[c],
Oathokwa Nkomazana, MB ChB, FCOpth (SA), MSc, PhD[d],
Victoria L. Williams, MD[b,e,*,1]

KEYWORDS

- Oculocutaneous albinism • Albinism • Quality of life • Botswana • Health care access • Stigma
- Discrimination • Disability rights

KEY POINTS

- Similar to populations with oculocutaneous albinism (OCA) in other regions, our cohort in Botswana faced difficulties obtaining equal rights to physical, psychosocial, and environmental health, contributing to lower quality of life (QOL).
- Skin health and visual impairment concerns, along with limited access to health care, created physical barriers to health for people with albinism (PWA) in Botswana.
- Psychosocial health was impacted by pervasive stigma and discrimination, along with myths and superstitions about albinism; these impeded social interactions and psychological functioning with negative emotions and thought/behavior patterns.
- Barriers to the successful personal development of education and employment, fears for safety, financial insecurity, and disability rights concerns created barriers to environmental health for PWA.
- PWA need disability rights protections to guarantee access to skin and visual health, equal opportunity for personal development, access to governmental support programs, and social inclusion to improve their overall QOL.

INTRODUCTION

Oculocutaneous albinism (OCA) is an autosomal-recessive disorder characterized by lack of melanin production in the skin, hair, and eyes.[1–8] Melanin is a pigment that absorbs ultraviolet light; hence people living with albinism (PWA) lack photoprotection and are more vulnerable to photodamage and skin cancers.[1,2,4,6–9] Because melanin-producing cells are critical for visual pathway development, all PWA have some level of visual dysfunction, which commonly includes nystagmus, strabismus, photophobia, and reduced visual acuity.[1,8]

The worldwide prevalence of the disease is approximately 1 in 17,000 births, with about 1 out of every 70 people carrying a gene for OCA.[1,2,8] However, OCA is more common in Africa, with prevalence rates of 1 in every 1000 births in some areas.[2,6,8,10] The risk of squamous cell

[a] Department of Dermatology, Perelman School of Medicine at the University of Pennsylvania, 2 Maloney Building, 3600 Spruce St, Philadelphia, PA 19104, USA; [b] Ministry of Health, Gaborone and Wellness, Headquarters, Private Bag 0038, Botswana; [c] Faculty of Social Sciences, Department of Psychology, University of Botswana, 4775 Notwane Rd, Gaborone, Botswana; [d] Faculty of Medicine, University of Botswana, 4775 Notwane Rd, Gaborone, Botswana; [e] Perelman School of Medicine at the University of Pennsylvania, 3737 Market Street, Philadelphia, PA 19104, USA
[1] Indicates a previous affiliation when this research was conducted.
* Corresponding author. 2 Maloney Building, 3600 Spruce St, Philadelphia, PA 19104, USA.
E-mail address: tori22@gmail.com

Dermatol Clin 39 (2021) 129–145
https://doi.org/10.1016/j.det.2020.08.012

carcinoma (SCC) has been reported as high as 1000 times greater in PWA in Africa than in the general population, and PWA are often diagnosed at advanced stages.[4,11] Reports have indicated that various social factors, such as poverty, low health care access, and limited knowledge about albinism, leave PWA vulnerable to higher rates of skin cancer and poorer outcomes.[2–4,7,11–14] Additionally, PWA in Africa face deeply embedded stigma, discrimination, and social marginalization, which can compound their health risks and affect quality of life (QOL).[2,7,9,15,16] A challenge unique to PWA in Africa is the widespread myths/superstitions that can drive persecution and murder of PWA for their body parts, which are used as talismans in African traditional medicine.[3,9]

QOL is defined as an individual's perception of their life in the context of their culture and value systems.[17,18] The World Health Organization (WHO) has emphasized the importance of QOL by defining health as the absence of disease along with a positive QOL.[17] QOL is strongly influenced by factors in an individual's physical, psychological, and sociocultural environments.[7,9,19] Assessing QOL is important for measuring the impact of disease on daily life to inform patient management and policy decisions.[16,18,20] Few studies have specifically investigated QOL for PWA, and thus far, poor health and social stigma are reported to detrimentally affect PWA in South Africa, Zimbabwe, Tanzania, Nigeria, and Brazil.[5,7,10,15,18,21] To the authors' knowledge, this is the first study to investigate OCA in Botswana, where epidemiologic data are lacking and local support programs for PWA are limited. By exploring the concerns with physical, psychosocial, and environmental health facing PWA throughout life, we aim to provide a baseline of information on the factors affecting QOL of PWA in Botswana, to illuminate strategies that can be undertaken to improve overall QOL in this population.

METHODS

We conducted qualitative semistructured interviews of PWA in Botswana. Participants were selected by convenience sampling from a larger cohort of 50 PWA older than 18 years old who were recruited from dermatology and eye clinics at Princess Marina Hospital or Tshimologo Albinism Association meetings in Gaborone, Botswana.

After informed consent, trained research assistants conducted interviews in participants' language of preference (Setswana or English) in a private room. A semistructured interview guide was used to explore issues of concern with life experiences across physical and mental health, education, employment, social interactions, and stigma/discrimination. Pertinent topics were decided based on literature review and author VLW's experiences working with OCA patients. Two pilot interviews (not analyzed in the results) were conducted to focus the interview guide. Additional interviews were conducted until saturation of themes was achieved. Interviews were recorded with consent and transcribed verbatim by research assistants.

QOL is complex and difficult to define, thus we chose to use a single framework outlined by the WHO for organizational structure.[17] The WHO breaks down QOL analysis into domains: physical, psychological, social interactions, and environmental health.[22] We combined social and psychological into one category because of the overlapping nature of topics covered.

Data were analyzed using the principles of thematic analysis.[23] Interview transcripts were uploaded onto MaxQDA software.[24] VLW read and reread the transcribed interviews and inductively developed codes from the data. EEA independently reviewed the data and developed codes. After rereading, both researchers agreed on final codes. Using the code family function, similar codes were grouped into categories based on identified relationships. VLW and EEA further interrogated the descriptive categories in the theoretic context of the WHO QOL domains and then agreed on overall categories to describe the data codes. Further interpretation and analysis of the categories led to the development of subcategories with themes to further describe the data that emerged from interview codes.

The study was approved by the institutional review boards of the University of Pennsylvania, University of Botswana, Princess Marina Hospital, and Ministry of Health and Wellness of Botswana.

RESULTS
Demographic Factors

Twenty-seven participants were interviewed with a male/female ratio of 1:1.6. The mean age was 37.9 (standard deviation, 14.7) with a range of 21 to 75 years old. All participants identified their ethnicity as Batswana.

Physical Health Factors

Skin health concerns
Every participant emphasized skin health as one of their greatest priorities in life, and many indicated a good understanding of the effects OCA had on their health: *"My skin easily gets burnt by the sun. If I do not protect myself I can get sores."*

(Participant [pt] 26). There was an understanding that engaging in sun protection was important to prevent the development of skin cancer: *"[Sun protection] is important because it prevents me from being killed by skin cancer."* (pt 36). Even more importantly, many participants understood the benefits of preventative measures in maintaining their health: *"It's very important to avoid sunburn. It is better to prevent than cure."* (pt 14).

Despite knowing the importance of sun protection, the degree to which participants understood how or were able to successfully protect themselves from the sun varied. Common methods for sun protection included clothing, shade structures, or staying indoors. However, a majority expressed difficulty in obtaining protective clothing because of finances or lack of availability in shops. Many felt helpless to avoid the sun because their activities of daily life, especially accessing transport and employment duties, required them to be outside: *"...I honestly think there is nothing I can do to improve sun-protection practices because I can't change the type of work I do, and I got other stuff to do for my life."* (pt 6). The lack of indoor employment opportunities created an internal struggle to balance their health needs with the need to earn money to support themselves: *"My jobs often require me to work outside, and I have no choice but to do it because I have to find some way to make money."* (pt 5).

Second to sun avoidance, sunscreen was described as the most important tool for sun protection and a central focus of participants' lives: *"I cannot live without sunscreen."* (pt 32).

"[Sunscreen] is a medication for us. It is life-saving, and we need it just like people need their blood pressure medications." (pt 8). However, nearly all participants faced challenges in obtaining an adequate supply of sunscreen including limited availability in pharmacies/shops, inability to reach places where it was available, inability to afford purchase, or dislike for the available sunscreen options.

Eye health concerns
One of the most common visual impairments associated with OCA is poor visual acuity and/or low vision, which can be significantly improved or corrected with appropriate treatment.[1,8,25,26] Participants universally indicated challenges in accessing refractive eye examinations and/or subsequently obtaining prescription eyeglasses. Although eye care and eyeglasses are covered through the public health care system in Botswana, rarely were participants able to obtain them. Health care system barriers included few

clinicians performing refractive examinations, one location with the equipment to make refractive lenses, and lack of supplies and/or technicians to produce eyeglasses. Nearly all participants lacked the finances to purchase eyeglasses or vision aids, and as a result, most had lived with some level of impaired vision.

Visual dysfunction had far-reaching consequences throughout participants' lives. Nearly all emphasized the direct effect visual impairment had on their education, indicating various barriers to successful learning summarized in **Table 1**. Participants lamented that low vision was the direct cause of their poor performance in school: *"If I had good vision I would not have failed like I did at school."* (pt 9). Additionally, low vision vastly narrowed employment opportunities, which were already limited by lack of education: *"Vision challenges really affect me because some jobs require a person with good vision, so I have no chance at these. Because of my poor vision I stay at home. I can't find work."* (pt 29). Navigating what would commonly be considered simple activities of daily life were fraught with challenges: *"getting around is a huge struggle. People don't realize how much of our society is set up against people with visual impairment. Why does there have to be glass doors? Why does there have to be shiny metallic windows or glass that reflects in all directions making it impossible for me to see without pain?"* (pt 7). Low vision often precluded participants from engaging in social activities, such as dancing, sports, or games that *"require one to have normal vision and play at a particular pace which I couldn't keep up because of my vision."* (pt 6).

The positive impact of successfully obtaining treatment to correct visual impairments was significant, resulting in some participants feeling their visual challenges were completely solved: *"I had problems with my vision when I did not have spectacles. When I had them, it was okay."* (pt 28).

Health care access challenges
Health care access is a complex and multidimensional topic that has been described to rely on the interconnected components of availability, accessibility, affordability, adequacy, and acceptability.[27] Although Botswana offers universal coverage to its citizens,[28] a unifying theme was that, despite attempts, participants faced difficulty in successful acquisition of health care. Barriers faced because of various health care access components are detailed in **Table 2**. One patient poignantly summarized her difficulty navigating

Table 1
Factors contributing to educational environments of people living with albinism in Botswana

Categories	Specific Factors	Representative Quotations (Participant Number)
Health-related barriers to learning	**Vision- related Challenges** • Difficulty seeing the board	• "I wouldn't see well, but if I come closer to the board, I was told that I distracted the other students…even though I understood Maths, I won't be able to see how the Math problems are solved to learn more and do well in the subject." (pt 35)
	• Difficulty writing on the board	• "…it was hard to write tests on the board with poor vision." (pt 10)
	• Difficulty reading (font size, color of fonts/background)	• "…reading small black letters on a white page was very difficult." (pt 26)
	• Difficulty using computers	• "I didn't continue with my studies because at tertiary…the types of computers were just not big enough for me to see and they would just tire my eyes." (pt 32)
	• Lack of materials for self-study	• "I had to wait for others to finish and borrow their books to write [notes]…sometimes they would refuse" (pt 10)
	• Time required to transcribe notes impeded time to learn	• "It made me to be behind with my school work because instead of revising I would be writing notes making me grasp little." (pt 10)
	• Not allowed extra time to complete assignments/tests	• "It was just hell. I was submitting my assignments late, I was finishing my tests late…. Teachers did not allow this so I was always in trouble." (pt 7)
	• Distracting eye pain (from straining, photophobia)	• "…when things were written on the board. I had bad eyesight…it would be painful." (pt 37) • "…there would be too much light into my eyes…and that would be painful." (pt 37)
	• Unable to access eyeglasses to correct low vision	• "My parents knew I was short sighted but we were [too] poor for them to buy me spectacles." (pt 45)
	Skin- related Challenges • Distracting skin pain (from sunburns)	• "For sure if the sun has really hit me, I cannot be able to go to school or to work." (pt 7)
Emotional barriers to learning	• Lack of confidence in their own intelligence	• "Ah! I was not smart enough that was the only challenge… I would have desire to learn but I would understand slowly." (pt 28)
	• Shame for not understanding their own educational needs	• "I couldn't tell my teachers that I can't see well because I was a kid and didn't really understand what was wrong. So I would write funny things and then later left school without giving reasons why because I was embarrassed." (pt 3)
	• Emotional distress from stigma-based bullying	• "So, I had to drop from school because of the teacher who was not treating me well. I would try to ask them to let me sit closer or make adjustments so I could learn better and the other kids would start teasing me. The teacher would tease me and start yelling." (pt 32)

(continued on next page)

Table 1
(continued)

Categories	Specific Factors	Representative Quotations (Participant Number)
Discriminatory barriers to learning	• Given lower priority in classrooms	• "Teachers did not give us the same opportunity as other kids. Even when we were better than them, they always got first priority. I think because they didn't want to deal with us and our poor vision..." (pt 33)
	• Teachers fear PWA	• "Some of the teachers were still afraid of us with albinism and so they were not making adjustments." (pt 13)
	• Teachers lack knowledge on needs of PWA	• "The teachers often have no knowledge about albinism or how to talk to the children, how to treat them, what they need, what visual problems they have..." (pt 32)
	• Teachers ignore bullying of other students	• "Some kids did not treat us well... I don't think teachers paid attention... I also did report to teachers, but they did nothing." (pt 45) • "...they would be spitting at me...it affected my ability to learn and to listen in class. Even if I would try to tell the teacher, she would be just ignoring this." (pt 21)
	• Teachers shaming/punishing for special needs	• "...even if I would ask the teacher to move forward they would say, 'No, no, no!' and they would scream at you and make you not have interest in going to school." (pt 32) • "Every time [I used the special needs bus transport], I would be like 20 or 40 min late and they [my teachers] would try to beat me [for being late to my class]." (pt 7)
	• Educational opportunities are held back	• "My parents did not want to take me to school because they believed I would not see written letters...Right now my age mates have achieved so much more in their life because of their education." (pt 14)
Resource limitations to learning environment	• Overcrowded classrooms	• "There were too many [students] in class and the teacher was not able to give me the attention and help I needed." (pt 31)
	• Teachers not trained for special needs of PWA	• "Some teachers were not trained to assist all students according to their need." (pt 10)
	• Limited or no access to special education programs	• "There was no special education, I was taught just like any other child who doesn't have albinism." (pt 5) • "I was going to a public primary school in Lobatse and they actually had a special needs department but I was not part of that. I tried to ask to be a part of that program, but they refused. They didn't see me as different from other people." (pt 7)

(continued on next page)

Table 1
(continued)

Categories	Specific Factors	Representative Quotations (Participant Number)
Positive changes to learning environment	• Teachers adjust learning environments	• "The teachers that did know would write on the board very large and in a dark color so that I could see. They would ask me where is it that I would be most comfortable, and I would tell them the front of the class and then that is, where I would sit." (pt 13)
	• Special education programs	• "When I was about to hit rock bottom...I found out there was a whole center dedicated to helping people like me with visual impairment. They taught me how to use visual tools, zoom text and JAWS. This made a huge difference in my education and allowed me to finish my studies successfully. But I can't help but wondering where was this unit for the first 2 y of my studies?" (pt 7)
	• Support from peers	• "At tertiary level I enjoyed my school days since my colleagues would not let me be alone. They would call me if I try to isolate myself and make me feel like I should be a part of the group." (pt 23)
	• Support from parents	• "My parents supported me and always informed my teachers to help me see better throughout my school days." (pt 23)

the public health care system in Botswana for treatment of a lip sore. Her care was delayed more than a year, resulting in the growth of a large nonoperable SCC of the lip (**Fig. 1**):

"They [the healthcare system] delayed to help me...but I used to come here [the hospital] daily...I first came when it [the skin cancer] was smaller...they kept doing tests and the results kept pending...and it grew bigger... I started at [my local clinic] who said should go to Oncology, and Oncology said I should go to Dental...then Dental said I should go back to Oncology to check if it is cancer. Because they wanted to do operation and the other doctors said you can't do operation without knowing the nature of the lesion, so go back to Oncology to do tests....It grew to this [size] before I was able to come to dermatology." (pt 9).

Psychosocial Health Factors

Stigma and discrimination

Participants reported a consistent onslaught of stigma and discrimination throughout life because of their outwardly identifiable genetic disease, resulting in a substantial negative impact on social interactions, employment, education, and

psychological health (**Table 3**). Albinism-associated stigma was experienced as feeling rejected, feared, isolated, "not human," "invisible," "diseased," or that they "do not exist." Discrimination was experienced as being made to feel of lesser value to others; socially excluded; and restricted in activities of daily living, education, and/or employment: "...*other people [make me] feel like I am nothing and I have no value.*" (pt 5). Many expressed an overall sense that society was "*avoiding trying to help us with albinism.*" (pt 29). Albinism-associated stigma was believed to even surpass the stigma of human immunodeficiency virus (HIV), which has been well-demonstrated as a major issue in Botswana society.[29–31]

Social interaction challenges

Stigma and discrimination created a clear impediment to the development of interpersonal connections associated with positive features of trust, respect, and esteem. From early childhood, some participants felt stigmatized and discriminated by their own families. Building and maintaining relationships with peers and romantic partners was strained. Interactions with members of society were fraught with unpredictable forms of harassment, marginalization, and restrictions. Even those who thought they found love and trust

Table 2
Health care access challenges for people living with albinism in Botswana

Health Care Access Challenge Categories	Challenges Faced	Representative Quotations (Participant Number)
Availability: *Do providers have the resources needed for diagnosis and management?*	**Limited availability of:** • Medications through government pharmacies • Equipment needed to treat the skin and eyes • Diagnostic tests leading to slow turnaround time • Specialist physicians in Botswana	• "Things like sunscreen, tablets… sometimes the hospital just doesn't have what I need." (pt 21) • "…today I came for cryotherapy but it was not there. So even when I can get to the clinic, it doesn't mean that I will be helped or that my problems will be fixed." (pt 45)

Accessibility: *Do patients struggle because of distance or time required to receive needed care?*	**Patients struggle with:**
	 • Navigating the multiple steps needed to get treatment
	 • Specialist appointments that are:
	   • Difficult to obtain Have long wait times
	   • Require long distance travel
		• "It took long for them [the health care system] to help me, but I used to come here [the hospital] daily…" (pt 9)
		 • "I live very far out…maybe 10–15 h so I need support to get transport to Gabs to see a dermatologist because there is no one in my area that can do skin checks…" (pt 13)
		 • "I think everywhere in our country …we struggle with waiting times…one time I had to live with a tumor for close to 6 mo before it could be operated on…" (pt 7)

Affordability: *Do patients struggle to pay for needed health care or health care–related items?*	**Patients are unable to afford:** • Purchasing medications (when not available through public health care system) • Sunscreen • Time off work for clinic visits • Transport to clinics/hospitals	• "…I live 50 km away from Gaborone, it costs me more than I have to get to Gabs to see the dermatologist." (pt 26) • "Although I know the health care is available it doesn't always mean that it is easy to access. I find it difficult to ask for time off from work as often as I need." (pt 7)
Adequacy: *Do patients feel satisfied with the health care provided?*	**Patients believe care is inadequate because they:** • Believe it is ineffective or futile • Prefer traditional medicine or religious cures • Are unhappy with treatment side effects • Family/friends do not agree with the treatments	• "…you start thinking to yourself 'ah i don't think the hospital helps. I don't need to go there'. [PWA] end up just giving up and maybe never going back. Or maybe they try other cures like from their church or family." (pt 7) • "For those in remote areas it can be the family members keeping persons with albinism from seeking help and getting to see their doctors." (pt 8) • "… I dread having to face getting my skin cut or sprayed [at the dermatologist]…people around you will try to talk you out of going to the doctor." (pt 7)

(continued on next page)

Table 2 (continued)		
Health Care Access Challenge Categories	**Challenges Faced**	**Representative Quotations (Participant Number)**
Acceptability: *Do patients trust providers and believe that care is in line with their cultural and social values?*	**Patients believe care is unacceptable because they:** • Experience stigma/ discrimination from providers • Experience societal stigma/ discrimination for needing medical care • Feel neglected by the health care system • Feel scared to have leave their village for health care	• "Most of the time nurses just brush us off when we present with sores to the local clinic. They make it seem normal and just give us calamine lotion and then we just get worse." (pt 33) • "You get labeled as 'always out sick'…that alone makes you not have the confidence to go to the hospital. So you end up missing the most important thing that can make a difference in your life…" (pt 7) • "An albino needs sunblock and spectacles just like an HIV positive person needs ARVs…because she [the health care system] does not take statistics of albinos [like is done for HIV], she is unable to provide them adequate health care." (pt 35) • "[PWA] might be scared to leave their own area…so in this way they are kept from getting proper health care." (pt 13)

in marriage could still face stigma from their partner: *"Albinism became an issue that broke apart my family… Out of nowhere [my husband] developed this problem with albinism and not only turned against me but turned my children against me. He said 'just know that all along I was just making you a favor. People like you don't get married'…"* (pt 32). Social stigma was strong enough to affect parents of PWA, evidenced by alarming reports of young mothers committing suicide after birthing a child with OCA (pt 8, 32). Practices of self-harm, abandonment, and even infanticide have similarly been described in families of PWA in other African countries.[32]

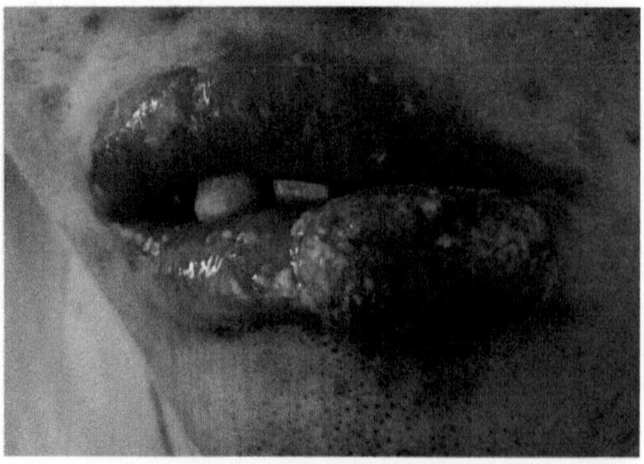

Fig. 1. Large invasive squamous cell carcinoma tumor of the left lower lip that grew during the course of diagnosis and treatment delays in a patient with albinism in Botswana.

Psychological impact

A cascade of negative psychological consequences developed from these experiences of stigma and discrimination (**Table 3**). Recurrent social rejection and lack of positive interpersonal experiences led to feelings of sadness, hopelessness, helplessness, resentment, fear, and shame typified by such sentiments as: *"I despise myself"* (pt 1) *and "what have I done to deserve this"* (pt 3). Negative thought and behavior patterns including low self-esteem, low self-efficacy, self-isolation, distrust, help-avoidance, and self-harm were common results. Some developed a habit of self-perpetuated negative thoughts that spiraled into a vicious cycle of learned helplessness, preventing participants from having enough self-efficacy to engage in measures to improve their life circumstances: *"As people with albinism, we internalize the hate others have for us and treat ourselves as worthless. How can we help ourselves when we don't see our lives worth living? When we don't think ourselves worthy of love and respect from others. In turn this makes us angry and resentful to others and this builds a viscous cycle of pushing people away and becoming more and more isolated."* (pt 7).

Table 3
Psychosocial impact of stigma and discrimination on people living with albinism in Botswana

Categories and Specific Challenges	Representative Quotations (Participant Number)
Social Interaction Challenges	
With Family	
• Not feeling accepted or supported by family • Restricted from family activities/events	• "... I would worry when discriminated by people at home where would I go and what would I do then...".[23] • "... within my husband's own family, even his sisters told me that we don't love you.".[8]
With Peers	
• Difficulty initiating and maintaining friendships • Exclusion from peer activities • Bullying from peers	• "Someone may have the desire to be my friend but then their family they don't accept me, and they force them to reject me.".[23] • "...I will be given a separate dish from others...my friends would tell me 'I can't eat with this one' or 'I can't sleep with this one' or 'I can't bath with this one' ...in many ways I would be singled out.".[35]
With Romantic Relationships	
• Difficulty initiating and maintaining relationships • Emotional bullying from significant others	• "It [albinism] is the reason why the father of my child is gone, because his friends will tell him 'how could he be with someone like this, why didn't you find a better person than this person with albinism.'".[29] • "Then he [my husband] came to me and said ... 'just know that all along I was just making you a favor. People like you don't get married. I did you a favor to marry you.'".[32]
With Society	
• Strangers avoid contact • Strangers react with fear and/or disgust • Verbal and/or physical aggression from strangers • Restricted from communal activities/events • Objectified as inhuman • Ignored when seeking help from societal/government institutions • Facing greater stigma than people living with HIV • Mothers of PWA react by inflicting self-harm • Stigmatized due to visible signs of medical treatment	• "When you try to greet someone, they act like they don't see you, like you do not exist.".[29] • "I experience [stigma] from the society... They despise and look down on us. Some act like we smell and sometimes spit saliva.".[45] • "When there are community works... I cannot participate... people do not want me to touch the food they eat.".[23] • "...we were told that we were not people, albinos are not human beings so we can't report mistreatment [at police stations].".[8] • "In government offices...they will say that they will be right back but then they never come back. It is clear that they are avoiding trying to help us with albinism.".[29] • "Being an albino is most discriminated than having HIV since some people are afraid of us, some feeling disgusted by our condition and we cannot hide it like you can with HIV....".[20] • "This past month there was a mom who committed suicide because she had a baby with albinism. You don't hear about that with HIV.".[8]
Employment Challenges	
• Excluded from opportunities to apply/interview • Denied employment offers	• "I was discriminated because of my skin color in jobs I have applied for...Eventually I only got

(continued on next page)

Table 3
(continued)

Categories and Specific Challenges	Representative Quotations (Participant Number)
• Fired without cause • Excluded from promotions • Bullied by coworkers/colleagues • Stigmatized for needing time off for health-care needs	a job because there was no one else [applying].".[30] • "Even colleagues that I have been working with for years, I hear them whisper about me. Saying I don't deserve the position I have.".[8] • "I find it difficult to ask for time off from work… I feel like others notice and keep track. It makes me feel diseased and like people feel that I am not as human because I need to see doctors so much.".[7] • "They stigmatize me by not letting me progress…They cannot give me a reason for why I do not get allowed to go for further training, they just give a reject to my requests.".[8]
Educational Challenges	
• See **Table 1**	
Psychological Impact Challenges	
Major Emotions: • Sadness • Hopelessness • Helplessness • Resentment • Fear • Shame Resulting thought/behavioral patterns: • Low self-esteem • Low self-efficacy • Self-isolation • Distrust of others • Help avoidance and denial • Self-harm/self-reproach • Self-perpetuated negative thought pattern	• "Yes stigma affects, it makes me feel sad and ask myself what wrong have I done to deserve this.".[3] • "I am sometimes hopeless…sometimes I wonder if I will manage. For example, when people are registering to receive government programs of poverty alleviation whereby we get goats. I do need them but I would wonder if I will manage them properly so in the end I don't end up even applying.".[36] • "I feel trapped like I cannot go where I want. Imagine you are not feeling well and you have no way to get to a doctor…You could even go to the bus stop and not know what routes to take. You feel isolated inside yourself because you are not exposing yourself to people and are hiding most of the time.".[32] • "So many people cocoon themselves because maybe they have been denied or failed so many times in the past and now they just give up. They don't even seek the resources or help that is, available.".[6] • "I even broke a bottle and stabbed myself to hurt myself because there was too much pain. I thought, 'If I wasn't like this with this skin…".[32] • "People with albinism just choose to suffer instead of standing up for themselves.".[8] • "We want things to change but…if people try to talk to us to bring change we are not so sure if it is real, you don't trust them and pressure keeps building and depression keeps building.".[7]

Myths and superstitions

Pervasive myths and superstitions associated with albinism emerged as additional negative contributors to psychosocial health. These included misinformation about how albinism is contracted and various beliefs about supernatural powers of PWA (**Table 4**). Participants reflected that these erroneous beliefs were likely fueling society's stigma/discrimination toward PWA. These beliefs also negatively contributed to the information participants had available to build their own self-concept. Particularly for children just learning about themselves, myths/superstitions seemed to impair their ability to develop a positive self-image and a sense of trust in others: *"It affected me because I didn't have any education about those myths. I didn't know if they were true or* *not when I was a child…. nobody was touching me or maybe one would run up to me and touch me just fast to see if the color could change. It made me very hurt. It made me feel that I was not a person. It was very tough."* (pt 21).

Environmental Health Factors

Participants discussed several factors affecting QOL in their external sociocultural environment, including issues with personal development, financial security, safety, and human rights.

Educational barriers to personal development

In addition to the vision-related barriers previously discussed, emotional barriers, discriminatory barriers, and resource limitations further compounded learning challenges for PWA (**Table 1**). Bullying

---

Table 4
Myths and superstitions about albinism in Botswana

Myths/ Superstition Categories	Specific Examples	Representative Quotes (Participant Number)
Myths about the humanity of PWA	• PWA are not human • PWA do not die • Men cannot truly love a woman with albinism	• "I hear people with albinism do not die but disappear." (pt 14) • "I hear them say all the albinos disappear and I felt insecure to hear that I disappear." (pt 35) • "When a man comes to a women with albinism he doesn't love her but he just wants to compare with a normal person or he is doing her a favor." (pt 8)
Myths about the contagion of albinism	• You must spit on yourself after seeing a PWA to prevent contraction of albinism • You will contract albinism by stepping where a PWA has been • Pregnant women who touch a PWA will give birth to a child with albinism	• "You have to spit on yourself when you see one to avoid becoming one." (pt 7) • "They say if you happened to stepped where an albino has stepped you're also going to change and you will have an albino child." (pt 21) • "The rumors I hear is that when you sit next to an albino and you are pregnant, you will give birth to a child like an albino." (pt 29)
Good luck superstitions	• Body parts of PWA can bring good fortune • Body parts of PWA cure diseases in African traditional medicine • PWA cannot contract HIV • Having sex with a PWA can cure HIV	• "People with albinism are harvested for 'muti' for traditional medicine and to bring good luck." (pt 20) • "I have heard of people using body parts of people with albinism for traditional medicine." (pt 26)
Bad luck superstitions	• The touch of a PWA brings bad luck • Families of PWA are cursed	• "People did not want me touching their food because they thought I was bad luck." (pt 7) • "Some would say our family is cursed to have a child like me." (pt 21)

Abbreviation: HIV, human immunodeficiency virus.

from peers was common, and teachers would ignore or even shame students trying to exert their needs. Participants overwhelmingly complained that their educational environments did not provide them with an equal opportunity to "learn properly." As a result, they often avoided school, performed poorly, or quit at a young age.

Even when special education resources were available, they were not readily accessible: *"I found out there was a whole center dedicated to helping people like me with visual impairment…. I think about how long I suffered needlessly when they had everything I needed but were unwilling to share it."* (pt 7). For those who could access educational support, the impact was immense. One participant was able to excel in a challenging tertiary educational program as a result of an adjusted learning environment provided by an expatriate teacher: *"That was the very first time that any teacher took notice of my impairment and tried to help. I was able to finish the program and pass because of his help. The other lecturers didn't think that I should be treated differently than the other students and in our country there is no laws that mandates anything for visual disabilities."* (pt 21).

Employment barriers to personal development

Participants expressed frequent frustration with an inability to develop meaningful careers. Many were only able to get jobs in menial labor or within the government's public works program that required them to work long hours outside being exposed to dangerous ultraviolet radiation.[33] Visual impairments and educational deficits surfaced as root causes precluding satisfying employment and a consequent improvement in life circumstances: *"My vision problems affected me in that I could be educated, have a job to live better if I was able to see enough to get through school."* (pt 1).

Successful employment was also hindered by stigma and discrimination (see **Table 3**). Employment options suitable for the low vision and sun sensitivity of PWA were lacking, and employers were unwilling to make allowances for special needs: *"when employers see that I cannot be outside, they do not even give me a chance at a job."* (pt 17).

For the few successfully employed participants, stigma and discrimination impeded enjoyment of work and limited opportunities for promotion within their fields: *"At work, some people do not like me. Some feel disgusted. Some would not even want to talk to me or sit next to me, all because of the color of my skin. It makes it hard to enjoy work or do my job well."* (pt 26).

Financial security concerns

Additional consequences of poor education and limited employment opportunities were lower socioeconomic status and poverty. Many were struggling to access basic needs, such as food, shelter, transportation, health care, and education for themselves and their families. Low income prevented purchase of adequate clothing and personal care products that could help maintain skin health and comfort. Inability to access welfare support was a common concern: *"My doctor once wrote me a letter to give to social worker so that I get monthly rations, but even to now I am unable to get this support. So I am left with only the P200 that my child gives me…"* (pt 45).

Safety concerns

A general sense of anxiety and fear permeated the lives of many participants, namely because of reports of ritual killings of PWA across Africa and concern that these attacks could also occur in Botswana. Participants felt *"always afraid"* (pt 1) to be alone, to travel freely, or go out at night: *"I feel unsafe thinking that, at any time, someone might want to kill me and use my body parts."* (pt 26). Others felt unsafe because of the stigma/discrimination directed at them and concerned that verbal abuse might turn into physical abuse. Some experienced minor physical aggression, threats of violence, persecution, and/or attempts at kidnapping, but our participants gave no reports of ritual murders.

Additionally, low vision made participants feel inherently unsafe in their environments. Many struggled to navigate daily activities: *"In the street …we don't feel safe to cross the road."* (pt 23). Without being able to clearly see their surroundings, participants felt at high risk for accidents and criminal violence: *"I was once attacked at night by thieves. I couldn't see them until they were right on top of me… It's dangerous."* (pt 32).

Disability rights issues

Botswana's government upholds the goals of improving social welfare and empowering disadvantaged groups through various welfare services and poverty eradication programs.[34] However, many participants reported an inability to access these services because of stigma/discrimination, difficulty navigating the process of application, or directly being denied: *"…it is not as easy as people who are old, in wheelchairs or pregnant because for us we get people saying "no you guys are lying you are just like us why would we give you preferential treatment…."* (pt 7).

At the time of this publication, Botswana has no specific disability rights in place and does not officially recognize PWA as disabled by law. As a result, participants often had difficulty deciding whether they considered themselves disabled and, thus, to which rights and protections they were entitled. Many believed albinism should be considered a disability to give special protections that could decrease the challenges faced throughout life: *"[Our biggest problem is] not being viewed as disabled and being forced to compete with the rest of society in day-to-day life. There are no protections in place to help us and we are no match for the world the way it is set up."* (pt 7).

However, there was significant trepidation around the word "disability" and concern that labeling themselves as disabled might, in some ways, lessen their already low status in society. To avoid stigma/discrimination, some participants expressed a desire to be seen and treated as normal: *"We are not having a disability. We are just like anyone else and we can do things like everyone else. This would help people to accept those with albinism as they are."* (pt 13). For some, there was a lack of understanding that disability rights legislations aim to increase equitable access to basic human rights and social inclusion to pave the way for less societal stigma/discrimination.

DISCUSSION

Our qualitative investigation of the life experiences of PWA in Botswana revealed that numerous intersecting physical, psychosocial, and environmental factors can contribute to lower QOL in this population (**Fig. 2**). These findings are consistent with the negative psychosocial impact of OCA reported in other African and South American countries.[5,7,10,15,18,21,35] There was significant overlap and interplay between QOL factors, indicating that negative influences and challenges can become compounded and multiply throughout life. An overlying theme connecting the issues faced by PWA was difficulty obtaining equitable rights and access within Batswana society.

Although health care access is a common problem across Africa,[36] Botswana positively stands out as a country that offers universal health care for citizens.[28] However, participants reported significant health challenges, indicating the need to improve practical access for PWA. Upscaling dermatology, oncology, and ophthalmology skills, currently only available at limited district/tertiary hospital levels, is critically needed for PWA. Sensitizing providers across Botswana to the special needs of OCA and giving PWA priority status as a vulnerable population within the health care system would allow more rapid and reliable access to needed care.

Participants primarily suffered skin and eye challenges, as has been reported in previous epidemiologic studies.[1,2,4,6–9] An understanding of their own health risks was not enough to prevent sun damage and skin cancers, because most faced barriers obtaining sunscreen/sun protective clothing and could not avoid daily sun exposure. Interventions to widely distribute sunscreen that is consistently available for free or a low cost are vital to give PWA a mechanism to protect themselves regardless of their required work/life activities. Sunscreen is included on Botswana's public medication formulary; however, limited supplies are available for the entire population. One of the authors (VLW) initiated a program to improve health care for PWA at Princes Marina Hospital through prioritized patient scheduling, obtaining equipment for skin cancer treatment, creating patient and provider education materials, organizing awareness events, and most importantly distributing free sunscreen with the support of Lady Khama Charitable Trust. However, this program only reaches patients who can access regular dermatology clinic visits. Outreach campaigns offering clinical care to underserved areas along with the distribution of durable shade devices and/or reusable ultraviolet protective clothing could augment skin cancer prevention in a cost-effective and sustainable way.[3]

Vision-related challenges were the most frequently emphasized issue, which had a negative impact across all three domains of QOL. Prior research in African OCA populations has indicated visual impairments are nearly completely correctable with prescription lenses or low-vision aids.[1] However, in Botswana, few participants were able to obtain the necessary health care services to achieve functional vision. Similarly, in neighboring South Africa, one study demonstrated that 85% of children with albinism were living with less than 30% use of normal vision.[9] Living with low vision from childhood to adulthood had far-reaching effects on education, employment, financial security, health care access, social interactions, safety, and the psychological well-being of participants. Visual disabilities effectively limited the opportunity of PWA to become active participants in society. The cost of extending low-vision support services and prescription eyeglasses to PWA is a small price compared with the benefits to be gained from lifting this population out of a lifetime of disability. Standing Voice, a well-established albinism support organization, has

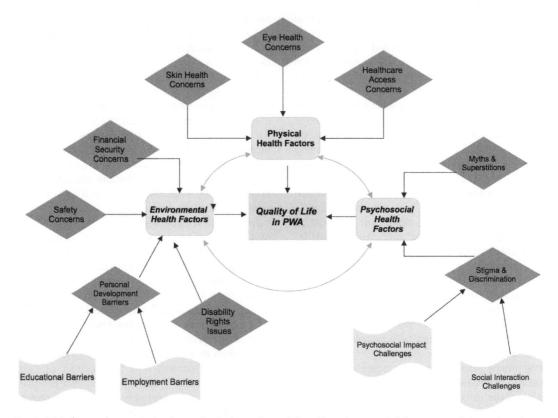

Fig. 2. This figure demonstrates how physical, psychosocial, and environmental factors can intersect and compound to contribute to lower QOL for PWA in Botswana.

developed a highly successful integrated skin cancer prevention and vision program in East Africa through partnerships with local governments and health care systems. Through large scale, rotating outreach clinics, they provide low-cost, on-site skin and eye care to hundreds of patients, dispensing up to 176 pairs of eyeglasses at a single outreach visit.[37] Their programs demonstrate the feasibility of high impact, scalable, and sustainable interventions for OCA health.

Psychosocial health is a cornerstone of QOL that is overlooked in developing countries facing more dire health crises, such as the HIV epidemic in Botswana.[38–40] However, without concurrently addressing psychosocial needs, interventions to increase the physical and environmental health of vulnerable populations may be less effective. Stigma and discrimination seemed to permeate all aspects of our participants' home/school/work and social lives. These effects have been similarly emphasized in other OCA studies.[2,5,7,9,15,16] Major psychological consequences included denial, self-reproach, and help avoidance behaviors, which could hinder efforts to support this population. Without the ability to feel safe, meet basic needs,

and feel supported/included within society, our participants neither felt worthy of accepting support, nor had the capacity to benefit society by reaching their true potential.

Environmental health factors of personal development, financial security, safety, and disability rights were also heavily influenced by stigma/discrimination and society's lack of awareness of the special needs of PWA. The educational system can provide early support for children to develop the skills needed to lead a productive and satisfying life.[5,7,41,42] Negative experiences commonly triggered PWA to discontinue school, and poor education is a known risk factor for several negative health and QOL factors.[41,43,44] There is untapped potential for interventions to improve educational outcomes for PWA in Botswana and other African countries. Widespread teacher education programs that emphasize identifying and adjusting to the needs of OCA students have been successful in Tanzania.[42] PWA can suffer lifelong consequences when they are not guaranteed the right to access education suitable for their special needs. Similarly, equal employment protections are needed to prevent the unfair challenges PWA face in obtaining safe and meaningful employment, a common struggle noted in surveys of PWA in other African countries.[16,18]

A repeated theme that summarized the intersecting factors contributing to low QOL was the viscous cycle that can trap PWA. It starts in childhood with visual dysfunction, leading to poor education combined with negative psychosocial interactions fueled by stigma and discrimination. Rare positive external influences trigger the development of a negative self-concept. Later in life, limited job opportunities caused by poor education and the physical limitations of OCA lead to higher rates of poverty. When jobs are obtained, the chance for upward mobility and success is thwarted by stigma/discrimination. Financial insecurity makes obtaining and maintaining health care more difficult. Because outside information is conflicting, PWA develop a sense of denial about their condition. There is confusion about whether they should fight for disability rights or fight to be "normal" citizens. Governmental support in the form of health care, social welfare, and disability services are available but, realistically, unattainable, suggesting efforts need to be made to assist PWA in understanding available programs and obtaining equitable access. Each time a participant's attempt at obtaining help was defeated, it encouraged a sense of helplessness and mistrust of society and its institutions. A dangerous sense of learned helplessness seemed to develop over time, encouraging PWA to effectively withdraw by not engaging in their own health care, personal relationships, or activities within their environments. Early positive and supportive influences in the lives of PWA would be key to prevent this negative path to low QOL. Models of successful OCA programs in other countries have used existing networks of OCA support groups as a means of disseminating education and linking individuals with support services to improve finances, education, health care, employment, and safety.[37,45] Because safety and trust was an expressed challenge in our cohort, we suggest interventions for PWA be implemented through groups with which they already feel a sense of connection and trust, such as OCA support groups, disability support groups, or religious groups.

In conclusion, our OCA cohort in Botswana faced similar challenges to PWA in other regions: a pervasive difficulty in obtaining equal rights to physical, psychosocial, and environmental health, which contributed to lower QOL.[2,3,7,10,35] Based on recommendations in the United Nation's Universal Declaration of Human Rights[46] and examples set by other African countries making strides in OCA rights, improving the lives of PWA in Botswana should start with ratifying disability rights protections and formally including OCA as a qualification for disability.[47,48] Currently, Botswana is 1 of only 11 countries on the African continent that have not ratified the United Nation's Convention on the Rights of Persons with Disabilities.[49] Significant efforts are needed to increase awareness and education on OCA across society, and institutions need legal support to help guide change. PWA need disability rights protections to guarantee access to skin and visual health, equal opportunity for personal development, access to governmental support programs, and social inclusion. The QOL framework we outlined could be used as a model to help explore the challenges and potential solutions for PWA in other regions globally.

Study limitations include the difficulty in generalizing results based on our convenience sample of participants engaged in positive societal activities (support groups or health care) in the capital city. Our results may differ compared with more isolated, rural communities in Botswana. Future studies should aim to investigate the prevalence, incidence, distribution, demographic features, and health outcomes of PWA, and triangulate our findings with quantitative QOL measures to improve understanding of this population.

CLINICS CARE POINTS

- Clinicians should be aware that visible skin diseases like oculocutaneous albinism can affect quality of life in a variety of ways that are dependent on local factors such as disability rights and cultural beliefs.
- To maintain skin health, clinicians should ensure patients with oculocutaneous albinism understand the risks of skin cancer and have access to sunscreen, sun protective clothing, and regular skin exams by a dermatologist.
- To prevent disabling visual dysfunction, patients with oculocutaneous albinism need yearly eye exams along with access to refractive lenses, low vision aids and other opthalmologic care starting from infancy.
- Parents and teachers should be aware that children with oculocutaneous albinism may face educational barriers due to health challenges, emotional challenges, discriminatory challenges and local resource limitations.
- Experiencing stigma and discrimination along with myths/superstitions about oculocutaneous albinism can have a far reaching negative psychosocial impact which can hinder a patient's engagement in their own healthcare.

ACKNOWLEDGMENTS

The authors are grateful for the support of the American Academy of Dermatology's Skincare in Developing Countries Grant which allowed Dr Williams to initiate a sunscreen distribution program for OCA patients at Princess Marina Hospital which has been sustained by the generous ongoing support of the Lady Khama Charitable Trust. We are grateful to Malebogo Ralethaka and Lesego Ndlovu for their contribution as research assistants in this study.

DISCLOSURE

The authors have nothing to disclose.

REFERENCES

1. Grønskov K1, Ek J, Brondum-Nielsen K. Oculocutaneous albinism. Orphanet J Rare Dis 2007;2:43.
2. Brocco G. Albinism, stigma, subjectivity and global-local discourses in Tanzania. Anthropol Med 2016; 23(3):229–43.
3. Brilliant MH. Albinism in Africa: a medical and social emergency. Int Health 2015;7(4):223–5.
4. Lekalakala PT, Khammissa RA, Kramer B, et al. Oculocutaneous albinism and squamous cell carcinoma of the skin of the head and neck in sub-saharan Africa. J Skin Cancer 2015;2015:167847.
5. Franklin A, Lund P, Bradbury-Jones C, et al. Children with albinism in African regions: their rights to 'being' and 'doing'. BMC Int Health Hum Rights 2018;18(1): 2.
6. Opara KO, Jiburum BC. Skin cancers in albinos in a teaching Hospital in eastern Nigeria: presentation and challenges of care. World J Surg Oncol 2010; 8:73.
7. Pooe-Moneymore MBJ, Mavundla TR, Christianson AL. The experience of people with oculocutaneous albinism. Health SA Gesondheid 2012; 17:1.
8. Wright CY, Norval M, Hertle RW. Oculocutaneous albinism in sub-Saharan Africa: adverse sun-associated health effects and photoprotection. Photochem Photobiol 2015;91(1):27–32.
9. Lund P, Franklin A. Albinism in East and Southern Africa knowledge based upon a descriptive literature review of research. Foundation of Applied Research on Disability; 2017.
10. Ajose FO, Parker RA, Merrall EL, et al. Quantification and comparison of psychiatric distress in African patients with albinism and vitiligo: a 5-year prospective study. J Eur Acad Dermatol Venereol 2014; 28(7):925–32.
11. Kiprono SK, Chaula BM, Beltraminelli H. Histological review of skin cancers in African albinos: a 10-year retrospective review. BMC Cancer 2014; 14:157.
12. Asuquo ME, Ebughe G. Major dermatological malignancies encountered in the University of Calabar Teaching Hospital, Calabar, southern Nigeria. Int J Dermatol 2012;51(Suppl 1):32–6, 36-40.
13. Lookingbill DP, Lookingbill GL, Leppard B. Actinic lentigines versus skin cancer risk in albinos in northern Tanzania. J Am Acad Dermatol 1995;33(2 Pt 1): 299–300.
14. Mabula JB, Chalya PL, Mchembe MD, et al. Skin cancers among albinos at a University teaching hospital in Northwestern Tanzania: a retrospective review of 64 cases. BMC Dermatol 2012;12:5.
15. Phatoli R, Bila N, Ross E. Being black in a white skin: beliefs and stereotypes around albinism at a South African university. Afr J Disabil 2015;4(1):106.
16. Baker C, Lund P, Nyathi R, et al, '. The myths surrounding people with albinism in South Africa and Zimbabwe. J Afr Cult Stud 2010;22:169–81.
17. Constitution of the World Health Organization. World Health Organization Handbook of basic documents. 1952;5:3-20.
18. Hong ES, Zeeb H, Repacholi MH. Albinism in Africa as a public health issue. BMC Public Health 2006;6: 212.
19. Patrick DL, Bush JW, Chen MM. Toward an operational definition of health. J Health Soc Behav 1973;14:6–23.
20. Guyatt G, Feeny D, Patrick D. Measuring health-related quality of life. Ann Intern Med 1993;118(8): 622–9.
21. Maia M, Volpini BM, dos Santos GA, et al. Quality of life in patients with oculocutaneous albinism. An Bras Dermatol 2015;90(4):513–7.
22. Programme on Mental Health. WHOQOL-bref survey manual. World Health Organization; 1996.
23. Braun V, Clarke V. Using thematic analysis in psychology. Qualitative Research in Psychology. 2008; 3;2: 77-101.
24. All-In-One Qualitative & Mixed Methods Data Analysis Tool. In: MAXQDA. 2019. Available at: www.maxqda.com. Accessed June, 2019.
25. Schulze Schwering M, Kumar N, Bohrmann D, et al. Refractive errors, visual impairment, and the use of low-vision devices in albinism in Malawi. Graefes Arch Clin Exp Ophthalmol 2015; 253(4):655–61.
26. Kirkwood BJ. Albinism and its implications with vision. Insight 2009;34(2):13–6.
27. Penchansky R, Thomas JW. The concept of access: definition and relationship to consumer satisfaction. Med Care 1981;19(2):127–40.
28. Tapera R, Moseki S, January J. The status of health promotion in Botswana. J Public Health Afr 2018; 9(1):699.

29. Letamo G. Prevalence of, and factors associated with, HIV/AIDS-related stigma and discriminatory attitudes in Botswana. J Health Popul Nutr 2003;21(4): 347–57.

30. Letshwenyo-Maruatona SB, Madisa M, Boitshwarelo T, et al. Association between HIV/AIDS knowledge and stigma towards people living with HIV/AIDS in Botswana. Afr J AIDS Re 2019; 18(1):58–64.

31. Wolfe WR, Weiser SD, Bangsberg DR, et al. Effects of HIV-related stigma among an early sample of patients receiving antiretroviral therapy in Botswana. AIDS Care 2006;18(8):931–3.

32. Kromberg J, Manga P. Albinism in Africa: historical, geographic, medical, genetic, and psychosocial aspects. London Academic Press; 2018.

33. Nthomang K. Botswana's ipelegeng programme design and implementation: reduction or perpetuation/entrenchment of poverty? Asian Journal of Social Science Studies 2018;3(3):27.

34. Republic of Botswana. Ministry of Local Government and Rural Development. In: GOV.BW. 2020. Available at: www.gov.bw/ministry-local-government-and-rural-development. Accessed April 29, 2020.

35. Masanja MM, Mvena ZSK, Kayunze KA. Albinism: awareness, attitudes and level of albinos' predicament in Sukumaland, Tanzania. Asian Journal of Applied Science and Engineering 2014;3(4): 382–95.

36. De Maeseneer J. Scaling up family medicine and primary health care in Africa: statement of the primafamed network, Victoria Falls, Zimbabwe. Afr J Prim Health Care Fam Med 2013;5(1):61–3.

37. Freeland H. Vision program. Standing Voice; 2018.

38. Brandt R. The mental health of people living with HIV/AIDS in Africa: a systematic review. Afr J AIDS Res 2010;8(2):123–33.

39. Geiselhart K. Stigma and discrimination: social encounters, identity and space; a concept derived from HIV and AIDS related research in the high prevalence country Botswana. 2009.

40. Gilbert L, Walker L. 'My biggest fear was that people would reject me once they knew my status…': stigma as experienced by patients in an HIV/AIDS clinic in Johannesburg, South Africa. Health Soc Care Community 2010;18(2):139–46.

41. Leino-Kilpi H, Johansson K, Heikkinen K, et al. Patient education and health-related quality of life: surgical hospital patients as a case in point. J Nurs Care Qual 2005;20(4):307–16 [quiz: 317–8].

42. Ndomondo E. Educating children with albinism in Tanzanian regular secondary schools: challenges and opportunities. Int J Educ Res 2015;3(6): 389–400.

43. Patti F, Pozzilli C, Montanari E, et al. Effects of education level and employment status on HRQoL in early relapsing-remitting multiple sclerosis. Mult Scler 2007;13(6):783–91.

44. Lasheras C, Patterson AM, Casado C, et al. Effects of education on the quality of life, diet, and cardiovascular risk factors in an elderly Spanish community population. Exp Aging Res 2001;27(3):257–70.

45. Freeland H. Skin cancer prevention program. Standing Voice; 2018. p. 1–58.

46. Human Rights Council. Independent expert on the enjoyment of human rights of persons with albinism. The United Nations. 2015. Available at: https://www.undocs.org/A/HRC/28/L.10. Accessed March, 2020.

47. General Assembly. Social development challenges faced by persons with albinism: report of Secretary-General. The United Nations; 2017.

48. Hillman A. Q&A: An International Movement for Albinism Rights. In: Voice by Open Society Foundations. 2019. Available at: https://www.opensocietyfoundations.org/voices/q-and-a-an-international-movement-for-albinism-rights. Accessed April 18, 2020.

49. Fernandez EL, Rutka L, Aldersey H. Exploring disability policy in africa: an online search for national disability policies and UNCRPD ratification. Review of Disability Studies: An International Journal 2019;13(1):1–12.

Integration of Management Strategies for Skin-Related Neglected Tropical Diseases

Lucinda Claire Fuller, MA FRCP[a,b,]*, Kingsley B. Asiedu, MD, MPH[c],
Roderick J. Hay, DM FRCP[b,d]

KEYWORDS

- Neglected tropical diseases of the skin ● Integration ● Mapping ● Training

KEY POINTS

- Neglected tropical diseases of the skin or skin NTDs: This is a new operational and strategic term used to describe those NTDs that have significant manifestations affecting the skin.
- Integration and NTDs: This approach allows health workers and policy makers to adopt common strategies and objectives for different diseases including diagnosis, treatment, and management of disability.
- Training and skin NTDs: Key to success of integrated approach is the development of effective training methods together with support networks to ensure sustainability.

INTRODUCTION

Neglected tropical diseases (NTDs) are a group of predominantly communicable diseases affecting the poorest and marginalized communities across the tropical and subtropical zones. The World Health Organization (WHO) list of NTDs includes 20 diseases affecting more than 2 billion people worldwide.[1] Although amendable to treatment or even elimination, they have been ignored by research and effective intervention and diagnostic strategies. Most of the diseases on the WHO list have recognized and significant skin manifestations and are known collectively as "skin NTDs."[2]

Disease that affects the skin in general is the third most common cause of all human illness affecting almost a third of the world population at any one time. Among these, fungal infections are the fourth most common of all illnesses and scabies, bacterial infections, eczema, and acne rank among the 50 most common of all human diseases.[3]

Skin disease is frequently highly symptomatic with disfigurement and unbearable itch being the most serious consequences of skin damage. Skin disease can also lead to long-term health complications and sequelae affecting other body systems, such as the heart, kidney, and joints. Additionally, the impact of skin disease on stigma and mental health is significant even leading to suicide.[4,5]

There has been a paradigm shift in medical policy and practice that now recognizes the benefits of pooling resources, coordinating efforts, and implementing collective actions, particularly in the discipline of tropical infectious diseases. Integration of NTD programs into the public health agenda has been a priority for global health over the past decade.

a Chelsea and Westminster NHS Foundation Trust, London SW10 9NH, UK; b The International Foundation for Dermatology, London W1P 5HQ, UK; c Department of Control of Neglected Tropical Diseases, World Health Organization, Geneva 1202, Switzerland; d The St John's Institute of Dermatology, King's College London, London SE1 9RT. UK
* Corresponding author. The International Foundation for Dermatology, London W1P 5HQ, UK.
E-mail address: claire.fuller@nhs.net

Dermatol Clin 39 (2021) 147–152
https://doi.org/10.1016/j.det.2020.08.013

WHAT ARE THE SKIN NEGLECTED TROPICAL DISEASES?

Skin NTDs include those NTDs that have recognized skin manifestations that are either primary manifestations of the disease, such as Buruli ulcer, leprosy, scabies, and mycetoma, or an associated clinical feature, such as the urticarial rash that can occur with schistosomiasis, soil-transmitted helminths, and foodborne trematodiases, or lymphedema that occurs with podoconiosis, and lymphatic filariasis (LF). Integrating approaches to NTDs may also crosscut with other noninfective chronic diseases; ulcer care in leprosy and diabetes mellitus is an example where an integrated approach provides benefits in terms of strengthening delivery of care and cost benefit.[6] Achieving global access to rapid diagnosis and control of these conditions and reduction in their associated stigma is a significant challenge but also a major opportunity.

Skin NTDs are not the only global health priorities with skin manifestations. Nonmelanoma skin cancer is the most common of all cancers, being the major occupational cancer presentation in many countries.[7] Chronic diseases, such as psoriasis, have significant impact on general health, particularly cardiovascular metabolic syndromes and mental health and life quality. This has been recognized in a World Health Assembly resolution (67.9). Human immunodeficiency virus/AIDS frequently presents initially with skin manifestations as the first sign of infection.[8]

Despite this case for a key role for dermatologic input, the demand for the knowledge and skills in diagnosing and managing skin disease outstrips the supply. There are limited training and research opportunities and poor access to effective medications that contribute to a large pool of inadequately or untreated patients.[9] Skin disease dominates patient presentations at the primary health care level, accounting for between 15% and 20% of primary care consultations, seemingly placing it in the front line for prioritization. Failing to address this situation is a major concern for those addressing health inequalities.

WHAT IS MEANT BY "INTEGRATION"?

Integration in this context refers to combining health care measures to address the detection and management of two or more diseases at the same time and in the same communities. Integration has the potential to be beneficial for several activities, from diagnosis and mapping to treatment and education.[10]

OPPORTUNITIES FOR INTEGRATION
Diagnosis

Several skin NTDs are coendemic in many areas of the tropics. Recognizing that skin disease is common, that skin manifestations are highly visible and contribute to stigma that further exacerbates the effects of poverty, offers an opportunity for a different approach. Skin disease is of considerable concern to patients, leading to their seeking attention if care is offered. This can facilitate community engagement in large-scale health intervention programs. Skin diseases are detected by visual examination so detection and even diagnosis may be provided by community health workers with basic training, potentially increasing patient access to health care and enabling early treatment.

Although the clinical signs of skin NTDs are varied, introduction of a simple syndromic method with an identification tool has been developed by WHO in the form of a training guide for health workers without specialist training to enable them to detect skin changes that may indicate an underlying skin NTD.[11] This tool focuses on four major skin changes: (1) ulcers, (2) lumps, (3) swollen limbs, and (4) patches. For each of these, a diagnostic flowchart leads the user to a likely diagnosis, possible treatment, and/or decision to refer on for specialist intervention.

The benefit of basic training for primary health workers to detect skin NTDs has been previously demonstrated in Mali. Focused, brief training sessions on the signs of leprosy and four other common skin diseases led to significant improvements in diagnostic accuracy, appropriateness of referrals, and the ability to effectively assess sensory function in patients with leprosy. This improvement was maintained when tested 12 to 18 months after the completion of the training compared with baseline.[12]

Traditional healers and practitioners of alternative therapies are commonly the first port of call for patients across many African countries and throughout India. They are popular, trusted by the community, and accessible. It has been shown to be feasible and cost effective to recruit and train these cadres to recognize and refer some diseases, such as leprosy, appropriately.[13–15] This showcases the importance of aligning any intervention in a way that is complimentary and supportive of the fragile health care systems providing for patients with skin NTDs.

A large-scale integrated, two-phased prevalence study in school children in Côte d'Ivoire found a sizable burden of skin disease affecting 25.6% of the 13,019 children screened. Superficial mycoses were the most common diagnosis and many children had two or more different skin diseases. With regards to skin NTDs identified, a single early case of leprosy and 36 cases of scabies were found.[16] Although this study offers a possible operational framework for the diagnosis and treatment of common skin disease and skin NTDs, it also illustrates the significant challenge this would pose in terms of demand on health services. Hypopigmented patches are far more likely to be pityriasis alba or versicolor rather than leprosy.[17] Similar experiences were reported from Benin, West Africa in an integrated control approach for Buruli ulcer, leprosy, and yaws. Using trained health care workers and community health volunteers, 15 cases of Buruli ulcer and three cases of leprosy were identified from the 1106 patients coming forward with skin disease. Although 185 cases of yaws were suspected, none were confirmed with point-of-care treponemal assay testing. Most cases were other skin conditions including fungal infections, eczema, and traumatic lesions.[18]

Single disease-based programs with a narrow focus may exclude the recognition and management of notable coexistent skin pathology, whereas an integrated approach to diagnosis enables the detection of multiple conditions at one time. The bulk of skin disease is accounted for by a few conditions, such as bacterial skin infections or pyoderma (impetigo and boils), superficial fungal infections, and noninfective conditions (eg, eczema and trauma); among the NTDs, scabies is also common. Applying simple algorithm-based detection and management schemes has been shown to be effective in various settings.[19,20] These provide an option for future integration efforts as an educational tool to upskill community health care workers in a rapid and appropriate way to diagnose and manage common skin problems.

Mapping

Disease mapping describes the gathering of geo-referenced data to depict the prevalence of a disease in time and space.[21] It uses geographic information systems that permit storage, analysis, and presentation of multidimensional data. Understanding detailed geographic distribution of skin NTDs is crucial for the planning of research and control strategies. High-quality epidemiologic data are lacking for many skin NTDs. Addressing this gap is a priority for developing the allocation of resources and intervention programs.

The publication of consensus diagnostic criteria available for skin NTDs without a point-of-care test, achieved now for scabies,[22] onchocerciasis,[23]

and podoconiosis,[24] has opened the way for combined mapping opportunities.

An excellent and early example of integrated mapping is provided by the African Program for Onchocerciasis Control.[25] Mapping of *Loa loa* distribution in the onchocerciasis endemic areas ensured that administration of ivermectin was avoided in *L loa*–coinfected communities. Ivermectin administration in patients with *L loa* is associated with a high risk of serious adverse events.

Combining mapping approaches across diseases with similar presenting features, demographics, and geographic predilections has been undertaken successfully for the common causes of lymphedema in the tropics. Podoconiosis is caused by prolonged contact with irritant volcanic red clay soils, and LF caused by infection with a parasitic nematode, *Wucheria bancrofti* (most commonly). Integrated mapping for LF and podoconiosis in Ethiopia has been successfully conducted across 659 districts over a 3-month period reaching 130,000 people from 1315 communities. LF was diagnosed by blood samples analyzing the presence of circulating *W bancrofti* antigen using an immunochromatographic card test. Podoconiosis was diagnosed clinically, having excluded other causes of leg swelling, such as onchocerciasis, leprosy, and rheumatic heart disease. Data were collected real time using smart phones and in-built global positioning system for the geographic coordinates.[26] After having reported the cost effectiveness and speed of this approach, further rapid integrated mapping has been undertaken across 20 districts in Ethiopia known to be coendemic for LF and podoconiosis to identify all lymphedema cases. Most (>95%) of the greater than 26,000 cases of lymphedema and/or hydrocele had leg lymphedema only, which could be attributable clinically to either LF or podoconiosis. The accurate mapping results are to be used to inform the morbidity and disability prevention planning process.[27]

Treatment

An approach to increase coverage for the seven most common NTDs (including the three major soil-transmitted helminths infections, schistosomiasis, LF, onchocerciasis, and trachoma), described as the "rapid impact package," combined the drugs for mass administration at a cost of $0.50 per person.[28] These packages included albendazole, praziquantel, ivermectin, diethylcarbamazine, and azithromycin. In addition to treating the seven main target diseases, additional infections covered therapeutically included strongyloidiasis, scabies, and other bacterial infections.

The so-called "off target" benefits of addressing symptomatic scabies, for example, contributed to community engagement with the process, because the reduction in itch experienced by the members of the community was popular.[29] Global Burden of Disease Study 2016 data have shown encouraging reductions in disease prevalence and burden (measured in disability-adjusted life-years) for six of the seven NTDs targeted by rapid-impact integrated mass drug administration (MDA) over the last decade.[30]

In addition to treating onchocerciasis, scabies, and strongyloidiasis infections, ivermectin is also effective against head lice and cutaneous larva migrans.[31] Integrated management can thus be achieved with this single drug.

The effectiveness and acceptability of ivermectin MDA for the management of scabies has been well documented and these data have, in part, led to the development of the World Scabies Elimination Program.[32,33]

However, a new agent related to ivermectin, moxidectin, a second-generation macrocyclic lactone with a longer half-life, is showing promising potential as a target drug for integrated MDA programs. It has been shown to be superior to ivermectin for onchocerciasis and trials are underway for establishing the correct dose for treating scabies.[34]

Morbidity Management

Although early intervention may achieve cure with minimal or no long-term sequelae, many skin NTDs lead to chronic health issues and a significant ongoing negative impact on quality of life. Skin NTDs producing lymphedema exemplify this well. Podoconiosis, LF, and even some deep fungal infections, such as chromoblastomycosis, induce significant and sometimes catastrophic lymphedema. Even when the infectious agent has been dealt with, in the case of LF and chromoblastomycosis, the lymphedema persists unless addressed. Simple hygiene-based management schemes for lower limb lymphedema with washing with soap and water, regular application of emollients, deep breathing and exercise, sleeping with the feet higher than the heart, bandaging, and wearing shoes have shown benefit in LF and podoconiosis.[35-37]

These water, sanitation, hygiene, and shoe-wearing approaches have also been shown to be of benefit in improving outcomes and reducing disease burden in other NTDs, such as trachoma (water, sanitation, and hygiene), schistosomiasis, soil-transmitted helminths, snake bites, tungiasis, and tetanus (shoe wearing). Integrated intervention packages around shoe wearing and care of the skin of the foot have great potential to benefit several skin NTDs, and improving outcomes for noncommunicable disease complications, such as diabetic foot ulcers. Are shoes the new "bed nets" for skin NTDs?

Skin NTDs lead to significant stigma and further exacerbate the suffering of affected individuals. The details leading to stigmatization across the different NTDs are alike; they include appearance, fear of contagion, being a burden to the family, and the inability to fulfill gender roles.[38] In some skin NTDs, such as leprosy, this has been exacerbated by discriminatory laws that further isolate affected individuals.[39] Integrated approaches to reduce stigmatization may be feasible and more efficient than disease-specific interventions. Understanding and measurement of the burden of stigma and disability is limited, but a toolkit shows promise in providing an integrated approach to addressing this challenge.[40]

Training

In addition to the WHO skin NTD Training guide for frontline health workers mentioned previously,[11] there are other educational tools that are addressing improving understanding of common skin diseases and their management and red flags for suspecting skin NTDs. The SkinApp produced by Netherlands Leprosy Relief is an algorithmic simple tool available via App Store or Google Play designed to support peripheral health workers in the recognition of the early signs and symptoms of skin diseases, including NTDs and skin manifestations of human immunodeficiency virus/AIDS.[41] Provision of specialist distance teaching or consultations through Telederm or WhatsApp-based programs is a further key measure to support front-line health workers.[42] The Community Skin Health Journal published by the International Foundation for Dermatology on behalf of the International League of Dermatologic Societies is a free dermatology resource for health care workers in underserved areas. It provides up to date, relevant information on the diagnosis and treatment of skin disease.[43]

Building the global health dermatology community to further support these training and intervention programs is underway with the establishment of the International Alliance for Global Health Dermatology (GLODERM).[44] Developing further collaborations across the Neglected Tropical Diseases Non-Governmental Organisations Network to ensure sharing of best practice and integration of interventions is also making progress with the launch of the Neglected Tropical Diseases Non-

Governmental Organisations Network Skin NTD Cross Cutting Group.[45] In addition, the International Foundation for Dermatology on behalf of International League of Dermatologic Societies coordinates global health partnerships that promote the understanding of skin health at the local, national, and international level.

SUMMARY

The grouping of skin NTDs provides a spotlight on the significant burden of skin disease that occurs mainly in impoverished populations in resource-poor settings. Building on the concept of skin NTDs smooths the path to integration of control activities from case acquisition, mapping, community empowerment, and treatment to disability and morbidity control. It enables clarification of the research gaps and priorities and supports a strong argument for funding to undertake further research and control activities.

Integrated control of skin NTDs led by the global health dermatology community and its partners has the potential to bolster health systems significantly and cost effectively in resource-poor areas, leading to improvements in skin health and overall health for many of the world's most disadvantaged individuals.[46]

DISCLOSURE

The authors have nothing to disclose.

REFERENCES

1. WHO list of neglected tropical diseases. Available at: https://www.who.int/neglected_diseases/diseases/en/.
2. Skin NTDs: the spectrum according to WHO. Available at: https://www.who.int/neglected_diseases/skin-ntds/en/.
3. Hay RJ, Johns NE, Williams HC, et al. The global burden of skin disease in 2010: an analysis of the prevalence and impact of skin conditions. J Invest Dermatol 2013;134:1527–34.
4. Dalgard FJ, Gieler U, Tomas-Aragones L, et al. The psychological burden of skin diseases: a cross-sectional multicenter study among dermatological out-patients in 13 European countries. J Invest Dermatol 2015;135:984–91.
5. Weiss MG. Stigma and the social burden of neglected tropical diseases. PloS Negl Trop Dis 2008;2(Issue 5):e237.
6. Puri V, Venkateshwaran N, Khare N. Trophic ulcers: practical management guidelines. Indian J Plast Surg 2012;45:340–51.
7. Fitzmaurice C, Abate D, Abbasi N, et al. Global, regional, and national cancer incidence, mortality, years of life lost, years lived with disability, and disability-adjusted life-years for 29 cancer groups, 1990 to 2017: a systematic analysis for the global burden of disease study. JAMA Oncol 2019. https://doi.org/10.1001/jamaoncol.2019.2996.
8. WHO guidelines on the treatment of skin and oral HIV-associated conditions in children and adults. Available at: https://www.who.int/maternal_child_adolescent/documents/skin-mucosal-and-hiv/en/.
9. Chandler DJ, Fuller LC. The skin: a common pathway for integrating diagnosis and management of NTDs. Trop Med Infect Dis 2018;3(3):101.
10. Integrating neglected tropical diseases into global health and development: fourth WHO report on neglected tropical diseases. Geneva (Switzerland): World Health Organization; 2017. Licence: CC BY-NC-SA 3.0 IGO Available at: https://www.who.int/neglected_diseases/resources/9789241565448/en/.
11. Department of Control of Neglected Tropical Diseases. Recognizing neglected tropical diseases through changes on the skin: a training guide for front-line health workers. Geneva (Switzerland): WHO; 2018. Available at: https://www.who.int/neglected_diseases/resources/9789241513531/en/.
12. Faye O, Hay RJ, Ryan TJ, et al. A public health approach for leprosy detection based on a very short term-training of primary health care workers in basic dermatology. Lepr Rev 2007;78:11–6.
13. Oswald IH. Are traditional healers the solution to the failures of primary health care in rural Nepal? Soc Sci Med 1983;17:255–7.
14. Kaur P, Sharma UC, Pandey SS, et al. Leprosy care through traditional healers. Lepr Rev 1984;55:57–61.
15. Ezenduka C, Post E, John S, et al. Cost-effectiveness analysis of three leprosy case detection methods in northern Nigeria. PLoS Negl Trop Dis 2012;6:e1818.
16. Yotsu RR, Kouadio K, Vagamon B, et al. Skin disease prevalence study in schoolchildren in rural Côte d'Ivoire: implications for integration of neglected skin diseases (skin NTDs). PLoS Negl Trop Dis 2018;12:e0006489.
17. Faye O, N'Diaye HT, Keita S, et al. High prevalence of non-leprotic hypochromic patches among children in a rural area of Mali, West Africa. Lepr Rev 2005;76:144–6.
18. Barogui YT, Diez G, Anagonou E, et al. Integrated approach in the control and management of skin neglected tropical diseases in Lalo, Benin. PLoS Negl Trop Dis 2018;12:e0006584.
19. Mahé A, Faye O, N'Diaye HT, et al. Definition of an algorithm for the management of common skin diseases at primary health care level in sub-Saharan Africa. Trans R Soc Trop Med Hyg 2005;99:39–47.
20. Steer AC, Tikoduadua LV, Manalac EM, et al. Validation of an integrated management of childhood illness algorithm for managing common skin conditions in Fiji. Bull World Health Organ 2009;87:173–9.

21. Brooker SJ, Smith JL. Mapping neglected tropical diseases: a global view. Community Eye Health 2013;26:32.

22. Engelman D, Fuller LC, Steer AC. International Alliance for the Control of Scabies Delphi Panel. Consensus criteria for the diagnosis of scabies: a delphi study of international experts. PLoS Negl Trop Dis 2018;12:e0006549.

23. Murdoch ME, Hay RJ, Mackenzie CD, et al. A clinical classification and grading system of the cutaneous changes in onchocerciasis. Br J Dermatol 1993;129:260–9.

24. Deribe K, Wanji S, Shafi O, et al. The feasibility of eliminating podoconiosis. Bull World Health Organ 2015;93:712–8.

25. Noma M, Nwoke BEB, Nutall I, et al. Rapid epidemiological mapping of onchocerciasis (REMO): its application by the African Programme for Onchocerciasis Control (APOC). Ann Trop Med Parasitol 2002; 96:S29–39.

26. Sime H, Deribe K, Assefa A, et al. Integrated mapping of lymphatic filariasis and podoconiosis: lessons learnt from Ethiopia. Parasit Vectors 2014;7: 397.

27. Kebede B, Martindale S, Mengistu B, et al. Integrated morbidity mapping of lymphatic filariasis and podoconiosis cases in 20 co-endemic districts of Ethiopia. PLoS Negl Trop Dis 2018;12:e0006491.

28. Hotez PJ. Mass drug administration and integrated control for the world's high prevalence neglected tropical diseases. Clin Pharmacol Ther 2009;85: 659–64.

29. Ndyomugyenyi R, Byamungu A, Korugyendo R. Perceptions on onchocerciasis and ivermectin treatment in rural communities in Uganda: implications for long-term compliance. Int Health 2009;1:163–8.

30. Hotez PJ, Fenwick A, Ray SE, et al. 'Rapid impact' 10 years after: the first 'decade'(2006-2016) of integrated neglected tropical disease control. PLoS Negl Trop Dis 2018;12:e0006137.

31. Ottesen EA, Hooper PJ, Bradley M, et al. The Global Programme to Eliminate Lymphatic Filariasis: health impact after 8 years. PLoS Negl Trop Dis 2008;2: e317.

32. Romani L, Whitfeld MJ, Koroivueta J, et al. Mass drug administration for scabies control in a population with endemic disease. N Engl J Med 2015; 373(24):2305–13.

33. The World Scabies Elimination Program. Available at: https://www.mcri.edu.au/research/projects/world-scabies-elimination-program.

34. Opoku NO, Bakajika DK, Kanza EM, et al. Single dose moxidectin versus ivermectin for *Onchocerca volvulus* infection in Ghana, Liberia, and the Democratic Republic of the Congo: a randomised, controlled, double-blind phase 3 trial. Lancet 2018;392:1207–16.

35. Stocks ME, Freeman MC, Addiss DG. The effect of hygiene-based lymphedema management in lymphatic filariasis-endemic areas: a systematic review and meta-analysis. PLoS Negl Trop Dis 2015; 9:e0004171.

36. Negussie H, Molla M, Ngari M, et al. Lymphoedema management to prevent acute dermatolymphangioadenitis in podoconiosis in northern Ethiopia (GoLBeT): a pragmatic randomised controlled trial. Lancet Glob Health 2018;6:e795–803.

37. Deribe K, Kebede B, Tamiru M, et al. Integrated morbidity management for lymphatic filariasis and podoconiosis, Ethiopia. Bull World Health Organ 2017;95:652–6.

38. Walker SL, Lebas E, De Sario V, et al. The prevalence and association with health-related quality of life of tungiasis and scabies in schoolchildren in southern Ethiopia. PLoS Negl Trop Dis 2017;11(8): e0005808.

39. International Federation of Anti-Leprosy Associations. Table of discriminatory laws. Available at: https://ilepfederation.org/discriminatory-laws/crimination/table-of-discriminatory-laws/.

40. Van 't Noordende AT, Kuiper H, Ramos AN, et al. Towards a toolkit for cross-neglected tropical disease morbidity and disability assessment. Int Health 2016;8:i71–81.

41. Mieras LF, Taal AT, Post EB, et al. The development of a mobile application to support peripheral health workers to diagnose and treat people with skin diseases in resource-poor settings. Trop Med Infect Dis 2018;3(3):102.

42. Williams V, Kovarik C. Long-range diagnosis of and support for skin conditions in field settings. Trop Med Infect Dis 2018;3(3):84.

43. Community Skin Health Journal. Available at: https://ilds.org/our-foundation/community-skin-health-journal/.

44. International Alliance for Global Health Dermatology. Available at: https://gloderm.org/.

45. Neglected Tropical Diseases NGO Networks Cross Cutting Groups. Available at: https://www.ntd-ngonetwork.org/cross-cutting-groups.

46. Engelman D, Fuller LC, Solomon AW, et al. Opportunities for integrated control of neglected tropical diseases that affect the skin. Trends Parasitol 2016;32: 843–54.

Printed and bound by CPI Group (UK) Ltd, Croydon, CR0 4YY

08/05/2025

01864700-0017